Machine Learning Approaches and Applications in Applied Intelligence for Healthcare Data Analytics

Innovations in Big Data and Machine Learning

Series Editors: Rashmi Agrawal and Neha Gupta

This series will include reference books and handbooks that provide the conceptual and advanced reference materials that cover building and promoting the field of Big Data and Machine Learning which will include theoretical foundations, algorithms and models, evaluations and experiments, applications and systems, case studies, and applied analytics in specific domains or on specific issues.

Artificial Intelligence and Internet of Things
Applications in Smart Healthcare
Edited by Lalit Mohan Goyal, Tanzila Saba, Amjad Rehman, and Souad Larabi

Reinventing Manufacturing and Business Processes through Artificial Intelligence
Edited by Geeta Rana, Alex Khang, Ravindra Sharma, Alok Kumar Goel, and Ashok Kumar Dubey

Convergence of Blockchain, AI, and IoT
Concepts and Challenges
Edited by R. Indrakumari, R.Lakshmana Kumar, Balamurugan Balusamy, and Vijanth Sagayan Asirvadam

Exploratory Data Analytics for Healthcare
Edited by R. Lakshmana Kumar, R. Indrakumari, B. Balamurugan, and Achyut Shankar

Machine Learning Approaches and Applications in Applied Intelligence for Healthcare Data Analytics
Edited by Abhishek Kumar, Ashutosh Kumar Dubey, Sreenatha G. Anavatti, and Pramod Singh Rathore

For more information on this series, please visit: https://www.routledge.com/Innovations-in-Big-Data-and-Machine-Learning/book-series/CRCIBDML

Machine Learning Approaches and Applications in Applied Intelligence for Healthcare Data Analytics

Edited by

Abhishek Kumar
Ashutosh Kumar Dubey
Sreenatha G. Anavatti
Pramod Singh Rathore

CRC Press
Taylor & Francis Group
Boca Raton London New York

CRC Press is an imprint of the
Taylor & Francis Group, an **informa** business

First edition published 2022
by CRC Press
6000 Broken Sound Parkway NW, Suite 300, Boca Raton, FL 33487-2742

and by CRC Press
2 Park Square, Milton Park, Abingdon, Oxon, OX14 4RN

© 2022 selection and editorial matter, Abhishek Kumar, Ashutosh Kumar Dubey, Anavatti G. Sreenatha, and Pramod Singh Rathore; individual chapters, the contributors

CRC Press is an imprint of Taylor & Francis Group, LLC

Library of Congress Cataloging-in-Publication Data

Names: Kumar, Abhishek, editor. | Dubey, Ashutosh Kumar, editor. |
Sreenatha, Anavatti G., editor. | Rathore, Pramod Singh, 1988- editor.
Title: Machine learning approaches and applications in applied intelligence
for healthcare data analytics / edited by Abhishek Kumar, Ashutosh Kumar
Dubey, Sreenatha G. Anavatti, and Pramod Singh Rathore.
Description: First edition. | Boca Raton : CRC Press, 2022. | Series:
Innovations in big data and machine learning | Includes bibliographical
references and index. | Summary: "In the last two decades, machine
learning has dramatically developed and is still experiencing a
fast and ever-lasting change in paradigm, methodology, applications, and
other aspects. This book offers a compendium of current and emerging
machine learning paradigms in healthcare informatics and reflects on the
diversity and complexity. Machine Learning Approaches and Applications
Applied Intelligence for Healthcare Data Analytics presents a variety of
techniques designed to enhance and empower multi-disciplinary and
multi-institutional machine learning research. It provides many case
studies and a panoramic view of data and machine learning techniques
providing the opportunity for novel insights and discoveries. The book
explores the theory and practical applications in healthcare and
includes a guided tour of machine learning algorithms, architecture
design, along with interdisciplinary challenges. This book is useful to
research scholars and students involved in critical condition analysis
and computation models"-- Provided by publisher.
Identifiers: LCCN 2021043556 (print) | LCCN 2021043557 (ebook) | ISBN
9780367676339 (hardback) | ISBN 9780367676346 (paperback) | ISBN
9781003132110 (ebook)
Subjects: LCSH: Medical informatics.
Classification: LCC R858 .M326 2022 (print) | LCC R858 (ebook) | DDC
610.285--dc23/eng/20211110
LC record available at https://lccn.loc.gov/2021043556
LC ebook record available at https://lccn.loc.gov/2021043557

ISBN: 978-0-367-67633-9 (hbk)
ISBN: 978-0-367-67634-6 (pbk)
ISBN: 978-1-003-13211-0 (ebk)

DOI: 10.1201/9781003132110

Typeset in Times
by Deanta Global Publishing Services, Chennai, India

Contents

Preface

This book is organised into 13 chapters. Chapter 1 deals with cellular senescence, which has emerged as a fundamental ageing mechanism that also contributes to diseases of late life, including cancer, atherosclerosis and osteoarthritis. Single-cell sequencing, especially RNA-Seq, has now delivered a step forward to understanding the diversity and function of subpopulations of cells. This new technology is an ideal approach to studying a systems-level problem like ageing as such experiments often generate big datasets for downstream integrative analysis.

In Chapter 2, the authors share a concept of growing interest in the clinical community in a new technique, photoacoustic imaging, and its possible clinical applications. One of the most prominent features of photoacoustic imaging is its ability to characterise tissue, leveraging differences in the optical absorption of underlying tissue components such as haemoglobin, lipids, melanin, collagen and water, among many others. In this review, state-of-the-art photoacoustic imaging techniques and some of the key outcomes pertaining to different cancer applications in the clinic are presented.

Chapter 3 deals with patient empowerment and also covers the indicators as well as outcomes and the impact of empowerment on the entire healthcare system. The increasing implementation of patient portals and their importance for health organisations by increasing convenience and service efficiency are elucidated. Since patient empowerment allows patient engagement in decision-making, it also provides an opening for the field of capacity building in rare diseases.

Chapter 4 deals with real-time artificial intelligence that is available for improved decision support and action planning in agriculture by implementing machine learning techniques to the Raspberry Pi board to control drones. Thus, the three goals of DAD (drones, agriculture and deep learning) are deep learning technology, agricultural activities, drone management and smart farming. This chapter concludes with a case study of applying the goals to urea spraying in the agricultural field. Furthermore, case studies can be made in other exciting fields of agriculture. The evaluation represents the different machine learning algorithms supporting the various agricultural sectors for more in-depth knowledge in the future.

In Chapter 5, the authors explain how clinical imaging has recently expanded lately because of the essential part it plays in medical service applications. Working along the lines of a natural eye, computer vision calculations discover examples and abnormalities in pictures to obtain a conclusion. Through a repetitive learning measure supported by neural networks, computer vision recognises, assesses and deciphers pictures.

In Chapter 6, the authors explain that although artificial intelligence helps people in general to improve, there are risks associated with its utilisation, set up in functioning frameworks, tools, calculations, framework the executives, morals and duty, and privacy. The study focuses on the risks and threats of computerised reasoning and how AI can help comprehend network safety or areas of cybersecurity issues.

In Chapter 7, the authors discuss privacy and security issues in multi-tenants in a single framework. For that problem, the artificial intelligence concept is used to improve the security and privacy concept in a multi-tenant-based system. Using artificial intelligence, the privacy and security concepts are made strong because in artificial intelligence work, as in intelligent human or animal minds, it takes maximum changes to fulfil the requirement of the concept to achieve the goal.

Chapter 8 provides detailed explanations of a novel approach for biometric recognition that has been introduced in which the application of ILBP (improved local binary pattern) for facial feature detection is discussed, which generates improved features for facial patterns. It allows only authenticated users to access a system, which is better than previous algorithms. Previous research on face detection shows many demerits in terms of false acceptance and rejection rates.

Chapter 9 explains how the developed system consists of a climbing robot, a camera for image capturing, IoT modules for transmitting images to the cloud, an image processing platform and an artificial neural network module intended for decision-making. The climbing robot holds a cable with grooved wheels along with the auto-trigger camera and the IoT module. For inspection, the robot ascends the cables continuously and acquires images of various segments of the cable. Then the captured images are sent to the cloud storage through an IoT system. The stored images are retrieved and their sizes are reduced through image processing techniques.

Chapter 10 deals with a robotic arm that is fixed to a base part consisting of wheels which are driven by DC motors. Lately, business and day-to-day schedule activities are discovered to be more alluring if carried out through mechanisation by means of robots. The identified spot mechanism is innovative, assembling businesses that are intended to perform pick and spot tasks. The framework was intended to such an extent that it disposes of human blunders and human intercession to achieve more exact work. There are numerous fields where human intercession is troublesome; however, a viable interaction must be worked and controlled, and this prompts the region wherein robots discover their applications.

In Chapter 11, the goal is to achieve secured communication through transmissions, and the received information is to be secured as there are chances of data hacking by unauthorised users. As the medium opted for in the communication process is wireless, there is also an online fraudulent threat of data. Due to these reasons, the medical data consisting of important patient details are secured and must be transmitted using error-correcting schemes for robust transmission as well. The algorithm that is chosen must be efficient and the channel must be reliable, promising the channel capacity achievement and retention of image quality with less distortion and low BER, which are the performance measures of the image transmission process.

Chapter 12 includes the multimodal and aspects of intelligent interaction along with the concept of how the novelty of HCI has come up by collaborating the usage of computers in this domain and thus has been named ambient intelligence. The chapter covers investigating the reliable factors that are responsible for adopting technical innovation through different models. According to the research, there are multiple factors on which individual adoption is indicated. This chapter attempts to illustrate the HCI and its state of the art towards its functionality and the factors that are responsible for the adoption of innovation for the improvement of the healthcare sector.

Chapter 13 provides an in-depth review of the administration of various techniques proposed by numerous researchers. A replacement system must be proposed which uses DL techniques and considers other attributes of paralysis agitans which can improve the prediction and be an advancement within the medical field. Result: it has been observed that many studies have identified the PD yet there is a need for a suitable method or algorithm to improve the prediction of PD which will help in clinical management. Conclusion and future work: most of the methods have used speech as a major attribute for their research and have produced substantial accuracy. In order to increase precision, approaches involving movements, facial expressions and other attributes should also be considered for evaluation.

Abhishek Kumar
Chitkara University Research and Innovation Network (CURIN)
Chitkara University
Punjab, India

Ashutosh Kumar Dubey
Department of Computer Science
Chitkara University
Punjab, India

Sreenatha G. Anavatti
School of Engineering and Information Technology
University of New South Wales
Canberra, Australia

Pramod Singh Rathore
Department of Computer Science and Engineering
University of Engineering and Management
Jaipur, India
and
Visiting Faculty
Maharshi Dayanand Saraswati University
Ajmer, India

MATLAB® is a registered trademark of The MathWorks, Inc. For product information please contact:
The MathWorks, Inc.
3 Apple Hill Drive
Natick, MA, 01760-2098 USA
Tel: 508-647-7000
Fax: 508-647-7001
E-mail: info@mathworks.com
Web: www.mathworks.com

Editors

Abhishek Kumar has a doctorate in computer science from the University of Madras and an MTech in Computer Science and Engineering from the Government Engineering College, Ajmer, Rajasthan Technical University, Kota, India. He has a total academic teaching experience of more than seven years with more than 80 publications in reputed, peer-reviewed national and international journals, books and conferences. He has guided more than 20 MTech projects and theses and is guiding two PhD scholars. His research area includes artificial intelligence, image processing, computer vision, data mining and machine learning. He has been session chair and keynote speaker at many international conferences and webinars in India and abroad. He has been the reviewer for IEEE and Inderscience journals. He has authored/co-authored six books published internationally and edited 16 books (published and ongoing with Elsevier, Wiley, IGI Global, Springer, Apple Academic Press, De Gruyter and CRC Press). He has been a member of various national and international professional societies in the field of engineering and research like a Senior Member of IEEE and IAENG (International Association of Engineers) and Associate Member of IRED (Institute of Research Engineers and Doctors). He received the Sir C. V. Raman National Award for 2018 in the young researcher and faculty category from IJRP Group. He is the editor of a special issue in the journal *Computers, Materials and Continua* (SCI and SCOPUS.IF-4.98), *Intelligent Automation and Soft Computing* (SCI, SCOPUS, IF-1.276) and *Cognitive Neurodynamics*, Springer (SCI, SCOPUS, IF-3.925).

Ashutosh Kumar Dubey is currently in the Department of Computer Science and Engineering, Chitkara University School of Engineering and Technology, Chitkara University, Himachal Pradesh, India. He received his PhD degree in computer science and engineering from JK Lakshmipat University, Jaipur, India. He is a Senior Member of IEEE and ACM. He has more than 14 years of teaching experience. He authored the book *Database Management Concepts*. He has been associated with many international and national conferences as a technical program committee member. He is also associated as an editor/editorial board member/reviewer of many peer-reviewed journals. His research areas are data mining, health informatics, optimisation, machine learning, cloud computing, artificial intelligence and object-oriented programming.

Sreenatha G. Anavatti is a Senior Lecturer with the School of Engineering and Information Technology at the University of New South Wales, Canberra, Australia. He has a PhD from the Indian Institute of Science, Bengaluru, India. Before moving to Australia, he was an Associate Professor at the Indian Institute of Technology, Mumbai, India. As an established faculty member at the Indian Institute of Technology, he has contributed to major national projects like the Indian remote sensing satellite, light combat aircraft and air-to-air missiles. His research work includes the application of AI for autonomous systems that include image processing for improved sensing and GAN-based networks for improved classification with imbalanced datasets. In addition, he also works on the application of modern control tools for applications related to aerospace, underwater and ground vehicles including evolutionary fuzzy and fuzzy neural systems for identification and control of dynamic systems. He has authored more than 250 papers in peer-reviewed international journals and international conferences. He has been an active reviewer for a number of high-quality journals like *IEEE Transactions* and a technical committee member for a number of international conferences such as SSCI.

Pramod Singh Rathore is pursuing his doctorate in computer science from the University of Engineering and Management (UEM) and has an MTech in computer science and engineering from the Government Engineering College, Ajmer, Rajasthan Technical University, Kota, India. He has been working as an Assistant Professor of Computer Science and Engineering at the Aryabhatt Engineering College and Research Centre, Ajmer, India, and also as visiting faculty at the Government University MDS Ajmer. He has a total academic teaching experience of more than eight years with more than 50 publications in reputed, peer-reviewed national and international journals, books and conferences such as Wiley, IGI Global, Taylor & Francis, Springer, Elsevier ScienceDirect, *Annals of Computer Science*, Poland, and IEEE. He has authored/co-authored six books published internationally and edited 16 books (published and ongoing with Elsevier, Wiley, IGI Global, Springer, Apple Academic Press, De- Gruyter and CRC Press). His research area includes NS2, computer networks, mining and DBMS.

Contributors

G. Aparna
Department of Electronics and
  Communications Engineering
Geethanjali College of Engineering and
  Technology
Hyderabad, India

P. Rupa Ezhil Arasi
Department of Computer Science
Muthayammal Engineering College
Namakkal, India

Rohidas B. Arote
Dental Research Institute
Seoul National University
Seoul, Republic of Korea

S. Arunmozhiselvi
Department of Computer Science and IT
DMI–St. John the Baptist University
Mangochi, Malawi

P. Manju Bala
School of Computer Science and
  Engineering
Nanyang Technological University
Singapore

Archana Chaudhary
Department of Biosciences and
  Environmental Science
SGT University
Gurugram, India

G. Glorindal
School of Computer Science and
  Engineering
Nanyang Technological University
Singapore

S. Iniyan
Department of Computing
  Technologies
SRM Institute of Science and
  Technology
Chennai, India

N. Jadhav
Department of Molecular Genetics
Seoul National University
Seoul, Republic of Korea

R. Jebakumar
Department of Computing
  Technologies
SRM Institute of Science and
  Technology
Chennai, India

M. Kezia Joseph
Department of Computer Science and
  Engineering
Usha Rama College of Engineering and
  Technology
Telaprolu, India

Yash Joshi
Department of Computer Science and
  Engineering
SRM Institute of Science and
  Technology
Chennai, India

G. Kalaimani
Department of Computer Science and
  Engineering
Shadan Women's College of
  Engineering and Technology
Hyderabad, India

G. Kavitha
Department of Computer Science and
    Engineering
Muthayammal Engineering College
Namakkal, India

T. Ananth Kumar
Department of Computer Science and
    Engineering
IFET College of Engineering
Gangarampalaiyam, India

Palvadi Srinivas Kumar
Department of Computer Science and
    Engineering
Usha Rama College of Engineering and
    Technology
Vijayawada, India
and
Department of Electronics and
    Communication Engineering
University College of Engineering,
    Osmania University
Telangana, India

Kesana Mohana Lakshmi
Department of Computer Science and
    Engineering
CMR Technical Campus
Hyderabad, India

Feng Lin
School of Computer Science and
    Engineering
Nanyang Technological University
Singapore

Sindhuja Manickavasagam
Department of Information Technology
Rajalakshmi Engineering College
Chennai, India

Neha Mehta
Chhattisgarh Swami Vivekanand
    Technical University
Bhilai, India

and
Department of Biosciences and
    Environmental Science
SGT University
Gurugram, India

Sachit Mishra
Department of Computer Science
    Engineering
SRM Institute of Science and
    Technology
Chennai, India

Vigneshwaran Pandi
Department of Computer Science and
    Engineering
SRM Institute of Science and
    Technology
Chennai, India

N. Prasath
Department of Computer Science and
    Engineering
SRM Institute of Science and
    Technology
Chennai, India

R.S. Ponmagal
Department of Computer Science
    Engineering
SRM Institute of Science and
    Technology
Chennai, India

Rishav Raj
Department of Computing
    Technologies
SRM Institute of Science and
    Technology
Chennai, India

Prabu Ramadoss
Dassault Systemes Austrila Private Ltd
West Perth, Australia

Tummala Ranga Babu
RVR & JC College of Engineering
Guntur, India

Jaiprakash Sangshetti
Quality Assurance
Y.B. Chavan College of Pharmacy
Aurangabad, India

Rituparna Singh
Department of Computer Science and
    Engineering
SRM Institute of Science and
    Technology
Chennai, India

R. Srivel
Department of Mechatronics
    Engineering
SRM Institute of Science and
    Technology
Chennai, India

S. Subha
Department of Computer Science and
    Engineering
Rajalakshmi Institute of Technology
Chennai, India

T. Tangarasan
Department of Computer Science and
    Engineering
KSR College of Engineering
Telangana, India

S. Usharani
School of Computer Science and
    Engineering
Nanyang Technological University
Singapore

S. Vani
Department of Mechatronics
    Engineering
SRM Institute of Science and
    Technology
Chennai, India

Ying Xu
School of Computer Science and
    Engineering
Nanyang Technological University
Singapore

1 Single-Cell RNA-Seq Technology for Ageing
A Machine Learning Perspective

Ying Xu and Feng Lin

CONTENTS

DOI: 10.1201/9781003132110-1

1

1.1 INTRODUCTION

1.1.1 DISCOVERY AND DETECTION OF SNCS (SENESCENT CELLS)

It was suggested by Hayflick in 1961 that normal human cells have a finite replicative capacity for cell division, which is a concept referred to as the "Hayflick
Limit". This finite proliferative capacity was now called replicative senescence.
This kind of senescence was thought to underlie the decline of cell replacement
and tissue repair that accompanies ageing and age-related diseases. This idea
was not able to be proven at that time as there were no methods to detect or
characterise in vivo.

Later, scientists found that senescent cells (SNCs) display β-galactosidase enzy-
matic activity at pH6. This β-galactosidase activity is now referred to as senescence-
associated β-galactosidase (SA-β-Gal) and this insight enabled the development of
a simple colourimetric assay now in widespread use for the labelling and detection
of SNCs. A second key tool was the identification of p16^{INK4A}, which is a cyclin-
dependent kinase inhibitor (CDKi) that functions as a master regulator of cell cycle
arrest in SNCs. Later, p19^{ARF}-mediated stabilisation of the transcription factor p53
was identified as a feature of SNCs, providing another valuable in vivo marker of
SNCs. These SNC detection tools as well as additional markers, such as accumulation of intracellular lipofuscin [1], established that senescence is a consequential in
vivo process and not merely a cell culture phenomenon. This can be depicted by the
cell cycle arrest in Figure 1.1.

1.1.2 CHARACTERISTICS OF SNCS

Our current knowledge of SNCs has been acquired largely using cell culture
systems, as the difficulties in detecting, tracking and collecting SNCs from aged
or diseased tissues mean that attempts to characterise SNCs in vivo have been
limited. From the research on SNCs, there are mainly three characters of them:

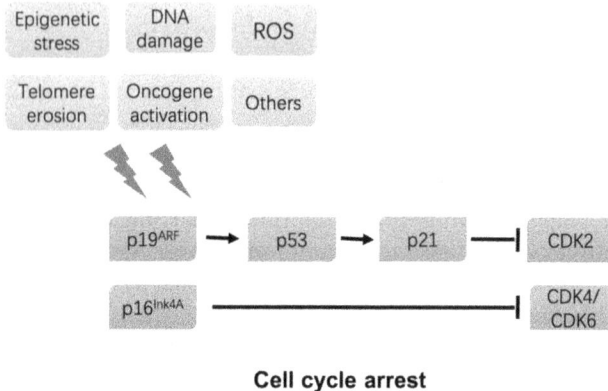

Cell cycle arrest

FIGURE 1.1   SNCs as a consequential in vivo process.

(1) First, SNCs are characterised by a state of permanent growth arrest that promotes organism survival by suppressing cancer. (2) Moreover, SNCs secrete a bioactive SASP (senescence-associated secretory phenotype) consisting of inflammatory cytokines, chemokines, growth factors and proteases. (3) SNCs show alterations in apoptotic signalling that, in general, cause resistance to programmed cell death. Computational models of Waddington's epigenetic landscape have been developed based on the dynamics of gene regulatory networks (GRNs). Our lab has developed a software tool called NetLand for modelling and simulating the kinetic dynamics of GRNs. By automating the modelling and visualisation of Waddington's landscape, NetLand can help analyse and predict the transcriptional regulation driving cellular phenotypic changes and explore the process of cell fate [2].

However, SNCs also possess beneficial functions which play an important role in preventing cancer and other biological processes. New technologies like systematic biological methods are required to help us understand the role of SNCs and thus develop therapeutic clearance of harmful SNCs. In this regard, supervised machine learning algorithms have been proposed and applied to answer biological questions concerning the underlying processes of ageing. Supervised machine learning findings support the link between ageing and longevity and specific types of DNA repair. The connections of age-related proteins between themselves and with non-age-related proteins were derived by supervised machine learning algorithms. It was shown that age-related proteins tend to be more connected than other proteins and also appear to be closer to each other in protein–protein interaction networks than other proteins. Several works have identified that autophagy/apoptosis-related proteins are related to ageing. Li et al. [33] classified human proteins as age-related or not using SVMs. They highlighted protein "VPS-34" as part of the autophagy process. Du et al. [34] proved that interactions with certain proteins like BLM, ATM, RPA1, PCNA and HSPA4, which are linked to the apoptosis of tumour cell lines, were good predictors of DNA repair age-related proteins. As the amount of age-related data increases, supervised machine learning tools have a greater potential to help experts studying the underlying process of ageing and senescent cells. In addition, this potential can be further explored with the combination of the predictions of supervised machine learning algorithms and wet-lab experimentation.

1.1.3 SNCs and Age-Related Diseases

Numerous age-related diseases have now been associated with cellular senescence, including cancer, atherosclerosis and osteoarthritis. The study conducted on a rapidly ageing animal (a mouse model with deficiencies in the mitotic checkpoint protein BUBR1 encoded by Bub1b) proved a link between SNCs and ageing. Experiments showed that the genetic inactivation of p16^{INK4A} blocked the formation of SNCs and attenuated the development of many ageing phenotypes, demonstrating that the accumulation of SNCs has been shown to trigger natural features of mouse ageing.

High-performance machine learning algorithms have been developed to discover interpretable knowledge [3, 4], for example, to find patterns to classify a protein as age-related or to investigate the importance of features used to predict the chronological age of individuals. Disorders in which SNCs have been implicated in disease may therefore be categorised according to whether SNC markers alone are used (SNCs correlate with disease), or whether prevention of cellular senescence or senolysis curbs or reverses disease (SNCs cause disease). In cases such as Alzheimer's disease and intervertebral disk degeneration, markers of SNCs are present in dysfunctional tissue, but there is no evidence for a causal role in disease pathogenesis [5]. However, this approach does not account for the non-SNC roles of these pathways and presumably blocks both SNC cell cycle arrest as well as SNC paracrine effects, such as the SASP.

Recent progress of therapeutic targeting SNCs includes senolysis (selectively eliminating SNCs), SASP neutralisation and immune-mediated SNC clearance. However, little is known about the actual senescence characteristics in various diseases, as our current methodologies require robust methods to retrieve and quantify SNCs in diseased tissue and we have limited molecular knowledge about these cells and their SASP profiles.

Machine learning methods predict candidate genes through various biological data, e.g. protein sequence, functional annotation, gene expression, protein–protein interaction networks, regulatory data and even orthogonal and conversation data. These methods are categorised as unsupervised, supervised and semi-supervised. Unsupervised methods cluster the genes depended on their proximity and similarity to the known disease genes and rank them by various methods. Supervised methods create a boundary between disease genes and non-disease genes, then use this boundary to select candidate genes [6]. Arabfard et al. designed a machine learning algorithm to identify and prioritise novel candidate ageing genes in humans. They made a binary classifier for predicting novel candidate genes upon the positively and negatively learned genes. They used three positive unlabeled learning (PUL) algorithms, Naïve Bayes (NB), Spy and Rocchio-SVM to evaluate the dataset and created a method for the isolation of human ageing genes from other genes. They identified reliable negative samples and tested the samples using a two-class classifier to identify novel positive ageing genes in humans.

With the advances in supervised machine learning algorithms, ageing has been studied at several levels of abstraction like the definition of the types of predictor attributes and the definition of the target variable. Some works use low-level features derived from "raw" amino-acid sequences of age-related proteins to define predictor attributes. Other works use biomarkers of higher-level biological systems like the metabolic and renal systems [7]. Some scientists even use non-traditional hierarchical features to represent instances, exploring the hierarchical relationships among gene functions available in curated ontologies like gene ontology (GO) [8]. Moreover, different types of target variables were used in ageing research like binary classification, hierarchical classification and regression. Machine learning plays an important role in ageing research and has even become effective in clinical prediction like for Alzheimer's disease.

1.2 MODELING OF CELLULAR HETEROGENEITY FOR DATA MINING

1.2.1 TRANSCRIPTIONAL NOISE

Gene expression in a biological process is shaped by various stimuli, thus noise can have cell-extrinsic or cell-intrinsic sources. Extrinsic noise is usually characterised by external signalling triggers, such as cell–cell or cell–matrix interactions, and chemokines that diffuse in the extracellular environment. Inflammatory signalling is also an extrinsic source of noisy expression. One example is that cells respond with oscillations in the production of NF-κB molecules and the downstream genes of the NF-κB pathway when triggered constantly by the cytokine TNF-α [9]. Extrinsic noise is shaped by the variability of extracellular signals and molecules, which are released from individual cells. Therefore, it is closely linked to intrinsic noise. Intrinsic noise stems from the inherent variability of intracellular and intranuclear fluctuations of molecules or alterations in the chromatin environment [10].

Another contributor to transcriptional variability is gene expression bursting, namely the stochastic activation and inactivation of transcription. These oscillations in transcription and translation are usually referred to as "bursts" because the production and degradation of molecules do not always follow the Poisson distribution. A recently published study on transcriptional burst kinetics demonstrates that the burst frequency and bursting size are actually encoded in core promoter elements and enhancers. They also reveal that burst kinetics play an important role in defining cell-type-specific expression patterns using allelic single-cell RNA sequencing. With the continued improvement of scRNA-seq technologies, it is now possible to precisely measure a minute amount of mRNA at the level of a single cell. Single-cell technologies for the first time makes it possible to measure genome-wide allelic patterns in a biological system and may enable the inference of global bursting kinetics.

1.2.2 CELLULAR HETEROGENEITY

Transcriptional noise and bursting both contribute to the heterogeneity of cells that are seemingly morphologically identical. Importantly, cell-to-cell variability can have profound effects on cellular function, as volume measurement of cells and tissue might mask these features. The recent development of single-cell sequencing technology has dramatically increased the resolution and sensitivity of heterogeneity measurements, which can even be applied in mixed cell populations [11]. Although this new technology overcomes limitations in bulk measurements and provides a high-resolution view of transitions among different cell states, the complexity of the data makes analysis and interpretation tough to achieve as well as the influence of factors on the heterogeneity of gene expression. Nevertheless, scRNA-seq has been successfully applied to identify unknown subpopulations of cells during transition stages in differentiation [12]. Buettner used a single-cell latent variable model (scLVM) to identify otherwise undetectable subpopulations of cells that correspond to different stages during the differentiation of naive T cells into T helper cells.

scRNA-seq enables the possibility to measure the heterogeneity in a pool of cells and capture cells at transition points during development and differentiation.

1.2.3 AGEING AND CELLULAR HETEROGENEITY

The question of increasing heterogeneity with age was proved by Philipp and his team [13]. They analysed various biophysical and biomolecular properties of cells. The effect of the cell cycle state can be observed in the biophysical properties of cells. The measurements indicated significant changes in cellular heterogeneity with age [13]. In addition, single-cell transcriptome analysis revealed a high degree of variability in mRNA level from cell to cell, indicating that one characteristic of senescent cells is higher transcriptional noise.

The first single-cell RNA dataset of aged cells was generated in cardiomyocytes in 2006. Fifteen genes were analysed by single-cell quantitative polymerase chain reaction (qPCR) in around 15 isolated cells each from young (six months) and old (27 months) mice [14]. The conclusion became clear that cell-to-cell variability was increased with higher age despite the limited data. This conclusion was consolidated by a study on around 2,500 single pancreatic cells, in which donor age spanned six decades. Noise clearly increased from young adults (21–22 years) to the mid-life span, suggesting that it would be even more profound at old age. In addition, gene expression alterations with increases in transcriptional noise have been reported to be associated with stress response genes like FOSB, HSPA1A and JUND, indicating that cellular stress might be important in the variability with age [15].

Recently, the data emerging from single-cell RNA-seq largely confirms the assumptions made in bulk experiments and indicates that ageing causes an increased cell-to-cell transcriptional variability, which might stem from general chromatin deregulation at older age [16]. In addition, published scRNA-seq data on CD4+ cells [17] with cell-to-cell epigenomic variability suggested that increased epigenomic noise is one mechanism that might lead to higher transcriptional noise with age. Taken together, these findings suggest that ageing is correlated with elevated cell-to-cell variability on an epigenomic and transcriptomic level and that these changes are supposed to be responsible for the cellular heterogeneity observed at a higher age.

Machine learning methods help specialists and biologists use functional or inherent properties of genes in the selection of candidate genes. Biologists apply computation, mathematics methods and algorithms to develop machine learning methods of identifying novel candidate disease genes. Scientists developed computational methods to predict biological age from gene expression data of tissue samples like skin fibroblast cells [18]. Horvath has applied the DNA methylation clock to categorise the age of human tissues and cell types. Similarly, Putin's deep learning method used blood cytology and chemistry to predict age [7]. Fleischer and his team suggest that skin fibroblast transcriptome data, coupled with machine learning techniques, can be a useful tool for predicting biological age in humans [18]. This progress also raised the possibility of developing a monitoring and prognostic tool for ageing and related diseases.

Normally, similar disease genes are likely to have similar characteristics. Some machine learning methods have been employed to predict new disease genes from known disease genes. Some computational machine learning approaches developed a binary classification model using known disease genes as a positive training set and unknown genes as a negative training set. These kinds of methods have been updated and improved and have become a promising way of predicting biological age.

With challenges in the single-cell sequencing, in order to specifically describe changes in the epigenome with transcript levels, both measurements would be performed in a single cell, which allows simultaneous measurements of DNA methylation and transcriptome.

1.3   MULTIMODAL SINGLE-CELL MEASUREMENTS FOR SAMPLE SEQUENCES

Initial single-cell technologies have focused on statistical modelling [19] and measurements of a single modality, for example, DNA sequence [20], RNA expression and chromatin accessibility [21]. In addition, ChIP-seq has become popular in the genome-wide study of protein–DNA interactions and histone modifications. We have invented a linear signal-noise model and developed an iterative algorithm, CCAT (control-based ChIP-seq analysis tool), to estimate the noise rate to represent the fraction of noise in a ChIP library [22]. Applications to H3K4me3 and H3K36me3 datasets showed distinct chromatin features associated with the strong and weak H3K4 me3 sites [23]. Although these technologies have yielded transformative insights into cellular diversity and development, this isolation limits the ability to derive a deep understanding of the relationships between biomolecules in single cells. Understanding the relationships is key to figuring out the cellular state and heterogeneity in ageing researches.

Recently, there has been some progress on the simultaneous profiling of multiple types of molecules within a single cell. This multimodal profiling can help build a more specific and comprehensive molecular view of the cell. Multimodal data can be obtained from single cells by four strategies.

1.3.1   THE APPLICATION OF AN INITIAL NON-DESTRUCTIVE ASSAY BEFORE SEQUENCING

As multiple scRNA-seq workflows utilise fluorescence-activated cell sorting (FACS), it is a natural extension to combine this single-cell isolation with index sorting to gather additional cytometric data about the cells before sequencing. This approach has been particularly successful in immunology and haematology, where well-defined cell surface markers are used to classify functional cell types and states or to discover rare cells in heterogeneous populations [24]. However, this kind of cytometric method can be limited by the spectral overlap between the fluorescent reporters.

1.3.2   SEPARATION OF DIFFERENT CELLULAR COMPONENTS
FOR PARALLEL EXPERIMENTAL WORKFLOWS

This strategy is especially useful for experiments aiming to simultaneously measure mRNAs alongside genomic DNA or intracellular protein in the same cell. Several groups have now achieved parallel genome and transcriptome sequencing from the same cell, which would allow direct comparison of genomic variation and transcriptome heterogeneity. Physical separation of mRNA and genomic DNA uses biotinylated oligo (dT) primers [25] and selective amplification of cDNAs over genomic DNA through in vitro transcription to achieve selective incorporation of T7 promoter sequences into cDNAs [26]. These methods will be of particular interest for tissues with high levels of genetic variation and chromosomal rearrangements, such as ageing.

Recent advances in scM&T-seq can sequence methylomes and transcriptomes from the same single cells [27], making it possible to reveal the complex relationship between DNA methylation and transcription in heterogeneous cell populations. As DNA methylation patterns are plastic and vary between different cell types, it is essential to decouple epigenomic variation from cell-type heterogeneity. Direct associations between epigenomic variation and transcriptional variation can be assessed by gathering DNA methylation and gene expression data from the same cell. In addition to between-cell analyses, scM&T-seq can also be used to correlate the methylome and transcriptome between genes in individual cells. scM&T-seq is a powerful approach to interrogate the poorly understood associations between transcriptional and DNA methylation heterogeneity in single cells and provides the potential to identify factors that regulate this relationship, which could become an important tool to study cellular heterogeneity in ageing.

Another advance in single-cell sequencing is the simultaneous collection of chromatin accessibility and gene expression data performed by selectively tagging genomic DNA and cDNA molecules with specific barcode sequences. Single-cell combinatorial indexing ("sci") methods use split-pool barcoding to uniquely label the nucleic acid contents of single cells or nuclei. sci-CAR, which jointly profiles single-cell chromatin accessibility and mRNA in a scalable fashion. sci-CAR effectively combines sci-ATAC-seq and sci-RNA-seq into a single protocol that could link the mRNA and chromatin accessibility profiles of individual cells. The sampling processes are depicted in Figure 1.2.

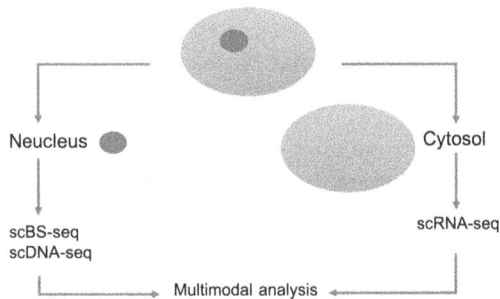

FIGURE 1.2   A single protocol linking the mRNA and chromatin accessibility profiles of individual cells.

1.3.3 Experimental Conversion of Multimodal Data into a Common Molecular Format

This conversion enables the simultaneous detection of multiple data types via a common methodology. For example, the simultaneous conversion of cell surface protein information and mRNAs into cDNAs allows both to be detected simultaneously via DNA sequencing. Two methods (CITE-seq and REAP-seq) exploit the use of DNA barcodes conjugated to antibodies to enable the measurement of cell surface protein abundance alongside mRNAs with single-cell resolution [28]. These methods circumvent some of the limitations of FACS-based cell surface protein detection through the utilisation of DNA barcodes to label antibodies. This progress allowed a more detailed analysis of single cells and enabled fine discrimination between immune cell types which was impossible with mRNA data alone. Extension of these methods using CRISPR-Cas9 provided unique opportunities to study the plasticity of cell fate [29].

1.3.4 Analysis of Different Data Types Encoded in Nucleotide Sequences

Although most scRNA-seq studies focus on transcript abundances, these studies can often provide information not just about transcript levels but also about nucleotide sequence, enabling multiple data modalities to be derived from standard scRNA-seq experiments without changes to experimental methods. Especially these possibilities include the capture of somatic mutations, genetic variants and RNA splice isoforms. Revealing the somatic mutations enables a more informative analysis of cancer biology and ageing.

Fan et al. devised a computational approach called HoneyBADGER to identify copy number variation and loss of heterozygosity in individual cells from single-cell RNA-sequencing data and applied their method to study multiple myeloma samples from patients, revealing transcriptional heterogeneity between cancer clones [30].

Single-cell analysis also offers a novel approach to understand how natural variation in DNA sequence influences variation in phenotypes such as gene expression and cell state. Kang et al. developed a computational tool, demuxlet, that use natural genetic variation to determine the sample identity of each droplet containing a single cell (singlet) and detect droplets containing two cells (doublets) [31]. Furthermore, they identified a genetic variant associated with altered proportions of immune cell types, highlighting the ability of this approach to model both gene expression and cell-type frequency as quantitative traits that can be associated with genetic variants.

Importantly, key information on transcript isoforms can be obtained from scRNA-seq data, even from methods that capture only the 3' end of gene transcripts. In addition, intron retention data can provide a large amount of information to complement transcript abundance measurements. By estimating the frequency of unspliced introns, scientists were able to predict the rate of change in transcript abundance and evaluate the future transcriptional state for each cell. Advances in these methods would transform the field of single-cell biology.

1.4 MACHINE LEARNING ON MULTIMODAL SINGLE-CELL DATA

1.4.1 ANALYSIS OF MULTIMODAL DATA

Although multimodal data analytical approaches are largely under development, for transcriptome [32], proteomics [33] and ChIP-seq [23], it is still a challenge to integrate different analytical approaches. Multimodal datasets are likely to reveal subtle differences in cell state that cannot be captured by a single modality alone. In some cases, other data from the same cells can fix the problem that incomplete detection of lowly expressed genes can blur fine-scale distinctions from scRNA-seq. Multimodal data of transcriptome and chromatin or methylation state may reveal heterogeneity in the regulatory landscape of individual cells.

Multimodal single-cell integration analytical approaches are inspired by many approaches, ranging from peptide alignments [34], biomarking for binding molecules [35] and MS/MS spectra analysis [36] to gene expression microarrays [37]. In particular, a multi-comics factor analysis (MOFA) method is capable of identifying a set of factors that explain variance from multiple data by analysing bulk genomic, DNA methylation and RNA expression data [38]. These researches reveal that methods are suitable for the analysis of multimodal single-cell data and may improve the explanation of the datasets in the future.

Multimodal single-cell experiments also offer a great opportunity to research the link between different components in a cell. For example, results of simultaneous mRNA and protein show poor relation, revealing active post-transcriptional regulation [28, 39]. A linear regression model which is built by Can et al. can predict gene expression values from chromatin accessibility data [40]. Regularised linear models have been built to evaluate the impact of a given set of guide RNAs in individual cells on gene expression levels. These methods detect that multimodal datasets are analysed by complex regulatory processes, including epigenomic, transcriptional and post-transcriptional gene regulation.

1.4.2 MACHINE LEARNING OF SCRNA-SEQ DATA

The Seurat v2 R toolkit first applies canonical correlation analysis (CCA) to calculate shared sources of variation between the datasets [41]. mnnCorrect depends on the identification of mutual nearest neighbours (MNNs), identifying cells that are closest to each other from different datasets [42]. CCA and mnnCorrect can integrate and pool scRNA-seq datasets from different laboratories and technologies on the same tissue. For elevating computational efficiency, Korsunsky et al. [43] developed a new variant of K-means clustering that is capable of integration of 500,000 cells on one personal computer, favouring clusters containing cells from multiple datasets.

Effective integration of single-cell datasets can far beyond batch correction and compare distinct biological conditions in depth at single-cell resolution. Butler et al. [41] identified 13 shared cell types between experiments and control groups from integration datasets of human peripheral blood mononuclear cells (PBMCs) across both control and interferon-beta-stimulated conditions by systematically comparing transcriptomes to identify cell-type-specific responses to stimulation. These analyses will find cell-type-specific responses to environmental and genetic perturbations.

The integration of scRNA-seq data also applies cross-species analyses as well. Karasikos et al. systematically compared expression profiles of orthologous genes across species and identify evolutionary changes [44]. Tosches et al. identified inhibitory subsets between the reptile and the mammalian brain [45]. At last, Alpert et al. developed cellAlign to compare scRNA-seq datasets of embryonic development between humans and mice [46]. All these methods remain at early stages. However, the accurate identification of gene orthologues across species is still a challenge.

1.4.3   CLASSIFICATION OF CELLS ACROSS scRNA-SEQ DATA

High-quality cell-type classifications will become more common. Scmap-cell and scmap-cluster are the related methods that project cells onto an existing dataset [47]. The scmap-cell identifies the nearest neighbours across datasets. The scmap-cluster classifies cells in a query dataset. The identification of cell subpopulations by reference-guided cell annotation can analyse closely related groups.

1.4.4   COMPUTATIONAL INTEGRATION OF MULTIMODAL SINGLE-CELL DATA

Cells from similar populations or common biological stats can be analysed across data modalities. For example, Welch et al. built a method, named MATCHER. This method is used to align different data types. They applied MATCHER to integrate scRNA-seq data with single-cell methylome and transcriptome (scM&T-seq) [27, 48] data during human induced pluripotent stem cell (iPSC) reprogramming.

Cell types are identified by the expression of cell-type-specific marker genes from scRNA-seq data. The cell-type-specific activity from other data modalities is less known. Lee JK et al. [49] performed single-nucleus RNA sequencing (snRNA-seq) and single-cell transposome hypersensitivity site sequencing (scTHS-seq) on a variety of matched brain tissue sections. The authors trained a model relating gene expression to chromatin accessibility. Similar methods can be used in the interpretation of single-cell DNA methylation or single-cell assay for transposase-accessible chromatin using sequencing (scATAC-seq) datasets.

Cross-modality classification of cells, as a new method, is developed. Welch et al. developed an integrative non-negative matrix factorisation (iNMF) method, named LIGER, which is capable of integrating data across modalities [49]. The authors also built an integration method, implemented in Seurat v3. This method assumes equivalent or correlated features in both modalities to classify cells across modalities [50]. These methods allow the identification of cell-type-specific patterns of chromatin accessibility and DNA methylation in different tissues.

1.5 PERSPECTIVES ON MACHINE LEARNING APPROACHES FOR AGEING

1.5.1 INTEGRATIVE AND LARGE-SCALE COMPUTATIONAL SYSTEMS FOR MACHINE LEARNING

Ageing is the time-dependent physiological functional decline in all aspects of a biological system, which ultimately leads to death. SNCs plays an important role in the ageing process. The investigation targeting SNCs is becoming an essential part of exploring the cellular changes during ageing and many senolytics were used to selectively eliminate senescent cells. However, as SNCs also possess beneficial functions like preventing cancer and other biological processes, how to analyse the complexities of senescent cells and selectively inhibit the negative effects without hurting the beneficial function still exists as the challenge in methodological innovations. From the perspective of the machine learning solutions [51], we have explored various architectural designs for high-performance computing [52] and embedded machine learning algorithms.

Along with the new machine learning method development, single-cell analysis techniques can combine computational modelling and simulation with large-scale experiments to explore dynamic behaviour in biological systems. Remarkably, the number of parameters that can be measured and the quantity of cells and molecules will increase, and large-scale collaborative efforts will enable us to build a comprehensive Human Cell Atlas. All these will require effective methods for data integration. Integration of RNA and DNA or protein is expected to be developed in the coming years. Studying the link between multimodal data types within individual cella will help us to understand the basis for cellular functions and infer causal relationships between modalities.

Specifically, computationally efficient unsupervised machine learning methods such as clustering [53] have been proposed. They can be applied to predict cell fate and age from the transcriptome of human cells in the classification of cell types. In the burgeoning use of single-cell data in clinical translational practice, accurate prediction of specific cell subtypes and age-related states will play an important role in the early diagnosis of age-related disease or informing personalised treatment. Along with the development of integration single-cell analysis and machine learning algorithms applied to automate the modelling and visualisation, wet-lab experiments to confirm the prediction and modelling are required. More potential can be further explored with the combination of the predictions of supervised machine learning algorithms and wet-lab experimentation.

1.5.2 A CASE STUDY: ORTHOGONAL VORONOI TREEMAP FOR UNSUPERVISED HIERARCHICAL CLUSTERING

The output of a data mining procedure can be adapted to two machine learning approaches: supervised classification (e.g. convolutional neural networks, CNN) of the samples if the domain-specific classes can be predefined and the class-labelled samples are available; otherwise, unsupervised clustering [54] of the samples without any domain-specific label. The latter, being an automated approach, is unable to classify the samples into the known knowledge subspaces, but can cluster the samples into their self-defined knowledge subspaces which can translate to knowledge discovery in domain-specific applications. In this case study, we propose an Orthogonal Voronoi Treemap (OVT) algorithm for unsupervised hierarchical clustering of complex data. The new algorithm will not only qualitatively describe the knowledge subspaces but also quantitatively divide the knowledge subspaces at different levels of hierarchy, as briefly introduced in the following.

Following the ageing knowledge representation scheme and SNC knowledge space boundary finding, we will partition the whole RNA-seq dataset into subregions based on distances to a set of points within the dataset. Briefly, given a bounded region Ω and a set of l sites $S = \{s_1, s_2, ..., s_l\}$, Ω is divided into a set of Voronoi cells $v(s_i)$, one for each site s_i. Then the cell $v(s_i)$ can be expressed as $v(s_i) = \{p \in \Omega \mid dist(p,s_i) < dist(p,s). \forall s \in S, s 6= s_i\}$, where $dist(p,s_i)$ is the distance between point $p = (x_p,y_p)$ and site $s_i = (x_{si},y_{si})$. In order to use the cells to depict data variants/measurements, a mechanism to control the areas of cells is required. Let $W = \{w_1, w_2, ..., w_l\}$ be a set of positive weights associated with the set of sites S correspondingly. Then the weighted power Euclidean distance can be written as $dist_{awpe}(p,s_i) = kp - s_ik^2 - w_i$, and the collection of Voronoi cells can be derived by $v(S) = \{v(s_1),...,v(s_l)\}$.

The proposed OVT is a recursive partitioning of the bounded region. Starting from the root of a hierarchy, a weighted Voronoi diagram is generated in the region Ω with one cell for each child of the root. An iterative optimisation process is taken to adaptively alert the value of the weight and the position of the site, such that the areas of the cells meet the requirement. The final layout requires that the area of each cell be in proportion to the associated measurements. If the area error reaches a threshold, the requirement is met and the iterative process converges. Therefore, let value si be the associated measurements of site s_i and let $E_{threshold}$ be the threshold of the area error; then the convergent requirement can be formulated, catering for domain-specific knowledge space.

We have also designed a Sweepline + Skyline strategy to fit the partitioning of orthogonal subregions. When the sweep line hits a new site, the relationship of this new site and all its site pairs are checked to generate vertical or horizontal segmentation lines. Meanwhile, a skyline is defined to record the current segmentation lines for all active sites. When the sweep line hits a new site and new segmentation lines are generated, the skyline will be updated correspondingly.

Experiments with the preliminary OVT algorithm have been conducted to verify the feasibility and repeatability in different datasets, as shown in Figure 1.3. It is found to be flexible to the changes of data measurements and can hold the nested orthogonal subregions to present each cell. Moreover, the OVT algorithm holds the stable aspect ratio in the treemaps. It preserves the relative positions of sites during iteration in order to visualise dynamic hierarchical data for which a more stable layout is essential. Verification on data transforms and preservations of radical relationships in hierarchical clustering have also been conducted.

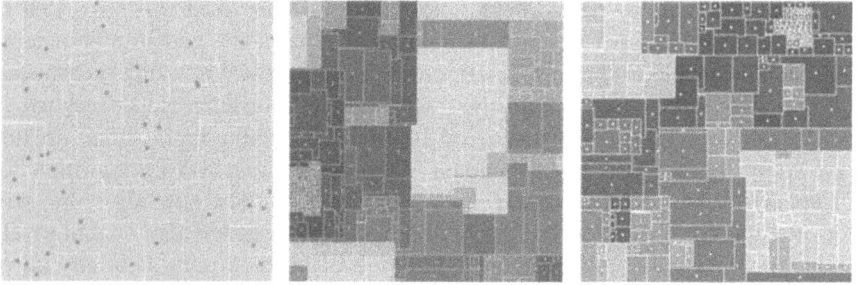

FIGURE 1.3 Preliminary OVT algorithm for hierarchical clustering of data points: (a) diagram of a series of random points, (b) OVT of the flare class hierarchy with random initial status, (c) OVT with the squarified treemap as initial status.

We have theoretically proven the new OVT algorithm with a time complexity $O(m \cdot \log[m])$ for m samples.

ACKNOWLEDGEMENTS

This work is partially supported by a grant (MOE AcRF RG93/20) by the Ministry of Education, Singapore.

REFERENCES

1. Evangelou K, Lougiakis N, Rizou SV, Kotsinas A, Kletsas D, Munoz-Espin D, Kastrinakis NG, Pouli N, Marakos P, Townsend P, et al: Robust, universal biomarker assay to detect senescent cells in biological specimens. *Aging Cell* 2017, 16(1):192–197.
2. Guo J, Lin F, Zhang X, Tanavde V, Zheng J: NetLand: Quantitative modeling and visualization of Waddington's epigenetic landscape using probabilistic potential. *Bioinformatics* 2017, 33(10):1583–1585.
3. Du Z, Lin F, Roshan UW: Reconstruction of large phylogenetic trees: A parallel approach. *Comput Biol Chem* 2005, 29(4):273–280.
4. Du Z, Feng L: pNJTree: A parallel program for reconstruction of neighbor-joining tree and its application in ClustalW. *Parallel Comput* 2006, 32:441–446.
5. Demaria M, O'Leary MN, Chang J, Shao L, Liu S, Alimirah F, Koenig K, Le C, Mitin N, Deal AM, et al: Cellular senescence promotes adverse effects of chemotherapy and cancer relapse. *Cancer Discov* 2017, 7(2):165–176.
6. Arabfard M, Ohadi M, Rezaei Tabar V, Delbari A, Kavousi K: Genome-wide prediction and prioritization of human aging genes by data fusion: A machine learning approach. *BMC Genomics* 2019, 20(1):832.
7. Putin E, Mamoshina P, Aliper A, Korzinkin M, Moskalev A, Kolosov A, Ostrovskiy A, Cantor C, Vijg J, Zhavoronkov A: Deep biomarkers of human aging: Application of deep neural networks to biomarker development. *Aging (Albany NY)* 2016, 8(5):1021–1033.
8. Chang J, Wang Y, Shao L, Laberge RM, Demaria M, Campisi J, Janakiraman K, Sharpless NE, Ding S, Feng W, et al: Clearance of senescent cells by ABT263 rejuvenates aged hematopoietic stem cells in mice. *Nat Med* 2016, 22(1):78–83.
9. Kellogg RA, Tay S: Noise facilitates transcriptional control under dynamic inputs. *Cell* 2015, 160(3):381–392.

10. Nikopoulou C, Parekh S, Tessarz P: Ageing and sources of transcriptional heterogeneity. *Biol Chem* 2019, 400(7):867–878.
11. Trapnell C: Defining cell types and states with single-cell genomics. *Genome Res* 2015, 25(10):1491–1498.
12. Buettner F, Natarajan KN, Casale FP, Proserpio V, Scialdone A, Theis FJ, Teichmann SA, Marioni JC, Stegle O: Computational analysis of cell-to-cell heterogeneity in single-cell RNA-sequencing data reveals hidden subpopulations of cells. *Nat Biotechnol* 2015, 33(2):155–160.
13. Phillip JM, Wu PH, Gilkes DM, Williams W, McGovern S, Daya J, Chen J, Aifuwa I, Lee JSH, Fan R, et al: Biophysical and biomolecular determination of cellular age in humans. *Nat Biomed Eng* 2017, 1(7): 0093. https://doi.org/10.1038/s41551-017-0093
14. Bahar R, Hartmann CH, Rodriguez KA, Denny AD, Busuttil RA, Dolle ME, Calder RB, Chisholm GB, Pollock BH, Klein CA, Vijg J: Increased cell-to-cell variation in gene expression in ageing mouse heart. *Nature* 2006, 441(7096):1011–1014.
15. Enge M, Arda HE, Mignardi M, Beausang J, Bottino R, Kim SK, Quake SR: Single-cell analysis of human pancreas reveals transcriptional signatures of aging and somatic mutation patterns. *Cell* 2017, 171(2):321–330.e314.
16. Booth LN, Brunet A: The aging epigenome. *Mol Cell* 2016, 62(5):728–744.
17. Martinez-Jimenez CP, Eling N, Chen HC, Vallejos CA, Kolodziejczyk AA, Connor F, Stojic L, Rayner TF, Stubbington MJT, Teichmann SA, et al: Aging increases cell-to-cell transcriptional variability upon immune stimulation. *Science* 2017, 355(6332):1433–1436.
18. Fleischer JG, Schulte R, Tsai HH, Tyagi S, Ibarra A, Shokhirev MN, Huang L, Hetzer MW, Navlakha S: Predicting age from the transcriptome of human dermal fibroblasts. *Genome Biol* 2018, 19(1):221.
19. Stepanova M, Lin F, Lin VC: Establishing a statistic model for recognition of steroid hormone response elements. *Comput Biol Chem* 2006, 30(5):339–347.
20. Stepanova M, Lin F, Lin VC: In silico modelling of hormone response elements. *BMC Bioinformatics* 2006, 7(Suppl:4):S27.
21. Xu H, Wei CL, Lin F, Sung WK: An HMM approach to genome-wide identification of differential histone modification sites from ChIP-seq data. *Bioinformatics* 2008, 24(20):2344–2349.
22. Han X, Lin F: *Computational Analysis of ChIP-Seq Data and Its Application to Embryonic Stem Cells* 2012. doi: 10.2174/97816080502531120101
23. Xu H, Handoko L, Wei X, Ye C, Sheng J, Wei CL, Lin F, Sung WK: A signal-noise model for significance analysis of ChIP-seq with negative control. *Bioinformatics* 2010, 26(9):1199–1204.
24. Paul F, Arkin Y, Giladi A, Jaitin DA, Kenigsberg E, Keren-Shaul H, Winter D, Lara-Astiaso D, Gury M, Weiner A, et al: Transcriptional heterogeneity and lineage commitment in myeloid progenitors. *Cell* 2016, 164(1–2):325.
25. Macaulay IC, Haerty W, Kumar P, Li YI, Hu TX, Teng MJ, Goolam M, Saurat N, Coupland P, Shirley LM, et al: G&T-seq: Parallel sequencing of single-cell genomes and transcriptomes. *Nat Methods* 2015, 12(6):519–522.
26. Dey SS, Kester L, Spanjaard B, Bienko M, van Oudenaarden A: Integrated genome and transcriptome sequencing of the same cell. *Nat Biotechnol* 2015, 33(3):285–289.
27. Angermueller C, Clark SJ, Lee HJ, Macaulay IC, Teng MJ, Hu TX, Krueger F, Smallwood S, Ponting CP, Voet T, et al: Parallel single-cell sequencing links transcriptional and epigenetic heterogeneity. *Nat Methods* 2016, 13(3):229–232.
28. Stoeckius M, Hafemeister C, Stephenson W, Houck-Loomis B, Chattopadhyay PK, Swerdlow H, Satija R, Smibert P: Simultaneous epitope and transcriptome measurement in single cells. *Nat Methods* 2017, 14(9):865–868.

29. Adamson B, Norman TM, Jost M, Cho MY, Nunez JK, Chen Y, Villalta JE, Gilbert LA, Horlbeck MA, Hein MY, et al: A multiplexed single-cell CRISPR screening platform enables systematic dissection of the unfolded protein response. *Cell* 2016, 167(7):1867-1882.e1821.

30. Fan J, Lee HO, Lee S, Ryu DE, Lee S, Xue C, Kim SJ, Kim K, Barkas N, Park PJ, et al: Linking transcriptional and genetic tumor heterogeneity through allele analysis of single-cell RNA-seq data. *Genome Res* 2018, 28(8):1217–1227.

31. Kang HM, Subramaniam M, Targ S, Nguyen M, Maliskova L, McCarthy E, Wan E, Wong S, Byrnes L, Lanata CM, et al: Multiplexed droplet single-cell RNA-sequencing using natural genetic variation. *Nat Biotechnol* 2018, 36(1):89–94.

32. Chen H, Mundra PA, Zhao LN, Lin F, Zheng J: Highly sensitive inference of time-delayed gene regulation by network deconvolution. *BMC Syst Biol* 2014, 8, Suppl 4(Suppl: 4):S6.

33. Li C, Li K, Li K, Lin F: MCtandem: An efficient tool for large-scale peptide identification on many integrated core (MIC) architecture. *BMC Bioinformatics* 2019, 20(1):397.

34. Du Z, Lin F: Pattern-constrained multiple polypeptide sequence alignment. *Comput Biol Chem* 2005, 29(4):303–307.

35. Rajapakse M, Schmidt B, Lin F, Brusic V: Predicting peptides binding to MHC class II molecules using multi-objective evolutionary algorithms. *BMC Bioinformatics* 2007, 8:459.

36. Li C, Li K, Li K, Xie X, Lin F: SWPepNovo: An efficient de novo peptide sequencing tool for large-scale MS/MS spectra analysis. *Int J Biol Sci* 2019, 15(9):1787–1801.

37. Han X, Sung WK, Lin F: Identifying differentially expressed genes in time-course microarray experiment without replicate. *J Bioinform Comput Biol* 2007, 5(2a):281–296.

38. Argelaguet R, Velten B, Arnol D, Dietrich S, Zenz T, Marioni JC, Buettner F, Huber W, Stegle O: Multi-omics factor analysis-a framework for unsupervised integration of multi-omics data sets. *Mol Syst Biol* 2018, 14(6):e8124.

39. Peterson VM, Zhang KX, Kumar N, Wong J, Li L, Wilson DC, Moore R, McClanahan TK, Sadekova S, Klappenbach JA: Multiplexed quantification of proteins and transcripts in single cells. *Nat Biotechnol* 2017, 35(10):936–939.

40. Cao J, Cusanovich DA, Ramani V, Aghamirzaie D, Pliner HA, Hill AJ, Daza RM, McFaline-Figueroa JL, Packer JS, Christiansen L, et al: Joint profiling of chromatin accessibility and gene expression in thousands of single cells. *Science* 2018, 361(6409):1380–1385.

41. Butler A, Hoffman P, Smibert P, Papalexi E, Satija R: Integrating single-cell transcriptomic data across different conditions, technologies, and species. *Nat Biotechnol* 2018, 36(5):411–420.

42. Haghverdi L, Lun ATL, Morgan MD, Marioni JC: Batch effects in single-cell RNA-sequencing data are corrected by matching mutual nearest neighbors. *Nat Biotechnol* 2018, 36(5):421–427.

43. Korsunsky I, Millard N, Fan J, Slowikowski K, Zhang F, Wei K, Baglaenko Y, Brenner M, Loh PR, Raychaudhuri S: Fast, sensitive and accurate integration of single-cell data with Harmony. *Nat Methods* 2019, 16(12):1289–1296.

44. Karaiskos N, Wahle P, Alles J, Boltengagen A, Ayoub S, Kipar C, Kocks C, Rajewsky N, Zinzen RP: The Drosophila embryo at single-cell transcriptome resolution. *Science* 2017, 358(6360):194–199.

45. Tosches MA, Yamawaki TM, Naumann RK, Jacobi AA, Tushev G, Laurent G: Evolution of pallium, hippocampus, and cortical cell types revealed by single-cell transcriptomics in reptiles. *Science* 2018, 360(6391):881–888.

46. Alpert A, Moore LS, Dubovik T, Shen-Orr SS: Alignment of single-cell trajectories to compare cellular expression dynamics. *Nat Methods* 2018, 15(4):267–270.

47. Kiselev VY, Yiu A, Hemberg M: Scmap: Projection of single-cell RNA-seq data across data sets. *Nat Methods* 2018, 15(5):359–362.

48. Welch JD, Hartemink AJ, Prins JF: MATCHER: Manifold alignment reveals correspondence between single cell transcriptome and epigenome dynamics. *Genome Biol* 2017, 18(1):138.

49. Lee JK, Wang J, Sa JK, Ladewig E, Lee HO Lee IH, Kang HJ, Rosenbloom DS, Camara PG, Liu Z, et al: Spatiotemporal genomic architecture informs precision oncology in glioblastoma. *Nat Genet* 2017, 49(4):594–599.

50. Stuart T, Butler A, Hoffman P, Hafemeister C, Papalexi E, Mauck WM, 3rd, Hao Y, Stoeckius M, Smibert P, Satija R: Comprehensive integration of single-cell data. *Cell* 2019, 177(7):1888–1902.e1821.

51. Du Z, Lin F, Schmidt B: Accomplishments and challenges in high performance computing for computational biology. *Curr Bioinform* 2006, 1(2):185–195.

52. Lin F, Schröder H, Schmidt B: Solving the bottleneck problem in bioinformatics computing: An architectural perspective. *J VLSI Signal Process Syst Signal Image Video Technol* 2007, 48(3):185–188.

53. Sasubilli SM, Kumar A, Dutt V: Improving health care by help of Internet of things and bigdata analytics and cloud computing. In *2020 International Conference on Advances in Computing and Communication Engineering (ICACCE)*, Las Vegas, NV, 2020, 1–4. doi: 10.1109/ICACCE49060.2020.9155042.

54. Kumar A, Sairam TVM, Dutt V: Machine learning implementation for smart health records: A digital carry card. *Glob J Innov, Opport Challeng AAI Machine Learn* 2019, 3(1).

2 Diagnosis in Medical Imaging
Emphasis on Photoacoustic Phenomena

*N. Jadhav, Jaiprakash Sangshetti
and Rohidas B. Arote*

CONTENTS

2.1 INTRODUCTION

Photoacoustic imaging (PAI) (Figure 2.1) is a developing imaging technique researched for various clinical applications, including oncology (Treeby et al., 2010), neurology, dermatology and ophthalmology (Kim et al., 2011). The strength of PAI lies in its ability to bridge the gap between pure optical and acoustic imaging, henceforth producing optical absorption-based images. Depending on the type of photoacoustic modality, PAI is able to achieve a resolution of submicrometres and reach a penetration depth that is as deep as several centimetres. The working principle of optical imaging methods is mainly governed by the scattering and absorption of photons, which can be categorised into four regimes. The ballistic regime is the region within the mean free path where the photons have not gone through any significant scattering. One example of an imaging system in this regime is confocal microscopy. In the quasi-ballistic regime, the region between the mean free path and the transport mean free path, the photons sustain minimal scattering. Nevertheless, this has a negligible impact on the photon's memory of the original path. Just below

DOI: 10.1201/9781003132110-2

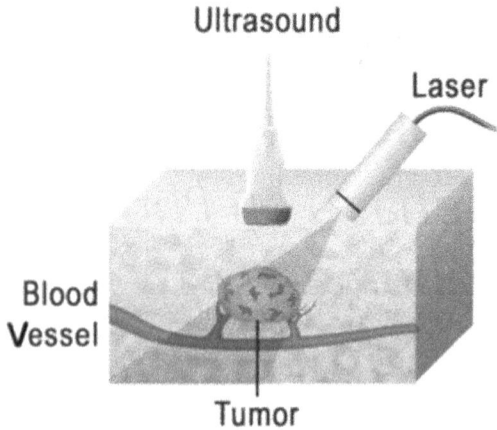

FIGURE 2.1 Principle of photoacoustic effect and imaging. When a tissue is exposed to a pulsed near-infrared laser, the tissue constituents such as haemoglobin, lipid, water, collagen, etc. absorb light and undergo thermoelastic expansion, thereby emanating ultrasound signals (photoacoustic effect).

the quasi-ballistic regime is the quasi-diffusive regime. In this regime, the photons are subjected to much scattering such that the spatial and temporal coherence is degraded. Beyond ten times, the transport mean free path is the diffusive regime. The photons in this regime have a negligible recollection of the original path. The spatial and temporal coherence is completely lost in this regime. For biological tissue, the mean free path is on the order of 0.1 mm while the optical transport mean free path is the order of 1 mm (Gambhir, 2012).

On the other hand, acoustic imaging makes use of the acoustic wave to penetrate deeper than optical imaging. Imaging is done based on acoustic contrast mismatch, which, in the case of biomedical imaging, is related to the mechanical properties of soft tissues. As acoustic impedance is not encoded with molecular information, therefore acoustic imaging is unsuited for monitoring molecular activities such as the oxygenation level in haemoglobin. Moreover, there is a trade-off between the penetration depth and the resolution where a high-resolution image commonly yields a low penetration depth and vice versa. This trade-off exists because the resolution produced by acoustic imaging is dependent on the frequency of the signal. A shorter pulse length is usually desirable as it gives a higher image resolution. However, with high frequency comes high ultrasonic attenuation. Consequently, it restricts the acoustic wave from penetrating deeper into the tissue.

Unlike acoustic imaging, PAI is able to take advantage of the optical contrast to provide histological, functional and metabolic imaging. Besides, in comparison to optical imaging, PAI does not need to take into account the scattering of the returning light and instead relies on the acoustic wave to form the image. This allows the PAI to produce optical absorption contrast images that cover beyond the quasi-ballistic regime. By detecting acoustic waves instead of photons, PAI has a depth-to-resolution ratio of two orders of magnitude higher than the common optical imaging methods. Furthermore, PAI is very sensitive to small changes in the optical absorption variation and can fully reflect these changes on the amplitude of the photoacoustic signal. This linear relationship between the signal and the optical absorption permits linear spectral unmixing for multiplex and functional imaging.

Employing the idea that every biological cell and tissue has different optical absorption coefficients, an appropriate wavelength can be selected for the specific target. Haemoglobin is one of the strongest optical absorbers in the visible light range. When a tumour develops in the body, the amount of blood flow in that region tends to be higher as more blood vessels grow to provide cancer cells with oxygen and nutrients. This is known as angiogenesis. With PAI, a specific wavelength, such as 532 nm, can be used to track haemoglobin. Thus, areas with high blood flow can be detected without exogenous labels. The ability to image haemoglobin will be immensely useful in aiding clinicians in the advancement of cancer studies. Other examples of endogenous contrast include melanin, lipids, and DNA/RNA. The absorption coefficient of some of the endogenous contrast at different wavelengths is shown in Figure 2.2. Exogenous contrast can be introduced to target specific cells or tissue when endogenous contrast is unable to produce a substantial signal. With a large variety of exogenous contrast available, selecting an exogenous contrast with a high absorption coefficient at the specified laser wavelength can improve the imaging sensitivity. Examples of exogenous contrast used in PAI are organic dyes, fluorescent proteins and nanoparticles.

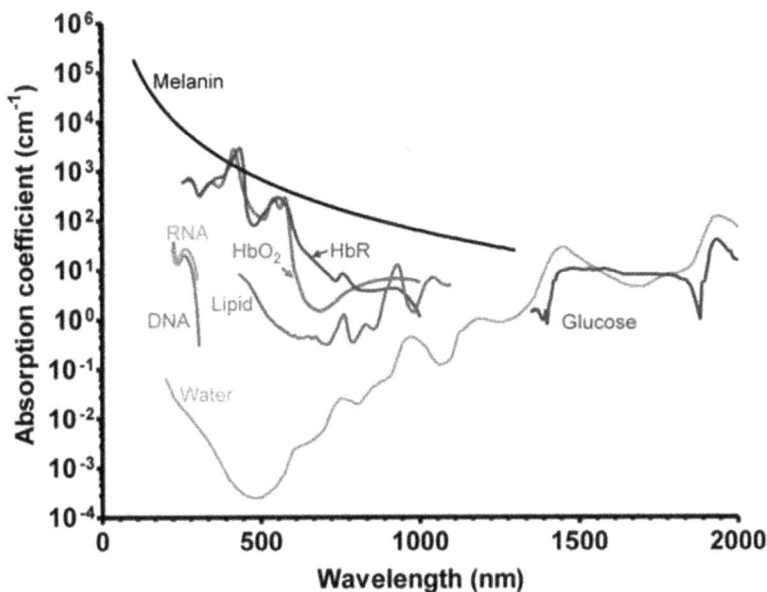

FIGURE 2.2 Absorption coefficient of various endogenous contrasts at different wavelengths. (From Heijblom, 2011.)

2.2   PHOTOACOUSTIC MODALITIES

PAI can be split into two main categories based on the way images are formed. Photoacoustic computed tomography (PACT) uses reconstruction-based image formation, while photoacoustic microscopy (PAM) uses focused-based image formation.

2.2.1   PHOTOACOUSTIC COMPUTED TOMOGRAPHY

In PACT, an unfocused optical beam is used to excite an area of the material, and an array of sensors measure the generated ultrasound waves in various positions. PACT has reportedly been able to penetrate as deep as 7 cm into tissue, but consequently, it may only deliver a lateral resolution of hundreds of micrometres. With different algorithms available, time reversal and back-projection methods are the two most popular techniques for image reconstruction. Time reversal is a time iterative reconstruction algorithm and, as its name suggests, works by re-emitting the wave in a time-reversed manner via an acoustic propagation model. Because of the intensive computation required to obtain the image, the time-reversal method has not been applied for practical use. The back-projection method, like time reversal, employs the knowledge of the speed of sound in the medium to resolve the ultrasound waves and back project them to form the image (Petrova et al., 2009). This method is similar to the delay and sum beamforming method used in ultrasound imaging. Since the back-projection method requires lesser time to form an image, it is more applicable for real-time imaging.

PACT can be used for many applications ranging from microscopic to macroscopic imaging. As it receives the signal from multiple elements, PACT can provide a larger field of view (FOV) with a single shot in the diffusive regime. Therefore, it can be used to image the whole body of small animals and has also been evaluated for uses in neurology, cardiology, and label-free breast cancer studies. However, imaging such a large field of view requires a large acceptance angle to receive signals from multiple locations of the same object. With such a large dataset, the imaging speed will be dependent on the data acquisition system.

2.2.2   PHOTOACOUSTIC MICROSCOPY

Unlike PACT, PAM uses a focused beam and detects using a single element that is raster-scanned about the sample. The signal which is dependent on the optical energy deposited is resolved with respect to the acoustic axis, and the envelope of this recorded time-domain signal is extracted to form the image. PAM is generally used for applications that require high-resolution images rather than deep penetration depth like the studying of the microenvironment of diseases using small animals. PAM can be further divided into two imaging methods depending on whether the generated photoacoustic signal is more optically or acoustically focused. Optical resolution photoacoustic microscopy (OR-PAM) takes advantage of the optical focus to obtain a high lateral resolution, while acoustic resolution photoacoustic microscopy (AR-PAM) utilises acoustic focusing to image at depths greater than the transport mean free path of the excitation pulse.

2.3 ACOUSTIC RESOLUTION PHOTOACOUSTIC MICROSCOPY

As mentioned previously, AR-PAM has a tighter acoustic focus for imaging. Since the acoustic focus is limited by the acoustic diffraction limit rather than the optical diffraction limit, the lateral resolution attainable by AR-PAM is only tens of micrometres. Conversely, acoustic waves scatter less than visible photons in scattering media. Hence, AR-PAM has been demonstrated to penetration depths of up to 11 mm, which is ten times more than OR-PAM.

The maximum permissible exposure (MPE) allowed by the American National Standard Institute (ANSI) for nanosecond pulsed wavelengths between 400 and 700 nm in human tissue is 20 mJ/cm2. As a larger area is illuminated, AR-PAM has a higher energy allowable limit than OR-PAM. This allows more photons to reach deeper into the tissue, producing higher quality images at deeper penetration depths. Moreover, AR-PAM is able to maintain the same contrast for a broad range of imaging resolutions. These advantages make AR-PAM a good imaging modality to be explored for different applications such as imaging sentinel lymph nodes detecting cystography, and gastrointestinal imaging.

2.3.1 OPTICAL RESOLUTION PHOTOACOUSTIC MICROSCOPY

OR-PAM, on the other hand, places emphasis more on the photons rather than the acoustic waves. In OR-PAM, the optical focus of the excitation beam is tightened to form the image. The lateral resolution is limited by the optical diffraction of the focused laser onto the tissue. Indeed, OR-PAM can produce images with higher lateral resolution than AR-PAM, but its penetration depth is restricted by the optical transport mean free path, which for biological tissue is ~1 mm (Liu et al., 2016).

Making use of its optical focus, OR-PAM can be used for label-free imaging within the optical quasi-ballistic regime. The high resolution that it can achieve makes it suitable for imaging small targets ranging from a capillary vein, which can be less than 10 μm, to even smaller targets like cells. OR-PAM has also been investigated for a broad range of applications to understand diseases and the biological environments in the eyes, skin and brain (Sivasubramanian and Pramanik, 2016).

2.3.2 DETECTORS USED IN THE DIFFERENT PAI MODALITIES

There are three detection geometries used in PACT applications, namely planar, cylindrical, and spherical. Planar view PACT systems usually use two-dimensional (2D) planar, phased, or linear arrays for imaging, while cylindrical view PACT systems detect with ring arrays. Spherical view PACT systems have been used for imaging with arc-shaped transducer arrays and hemispherical transducer 10 arrays. The axial resolution of all three PACT systems is determined by the bandwidth of the detector, while their lateral resolution is dependent on their detection geometries. Similarly, the axial resolution of PAM is also determined by the bandwidth of the detector; however, the lateral resolution is based on the acoustic wavelength for AR-PAM and the optical wavelength for OR-PAM. OR-PAM mainly relies on the

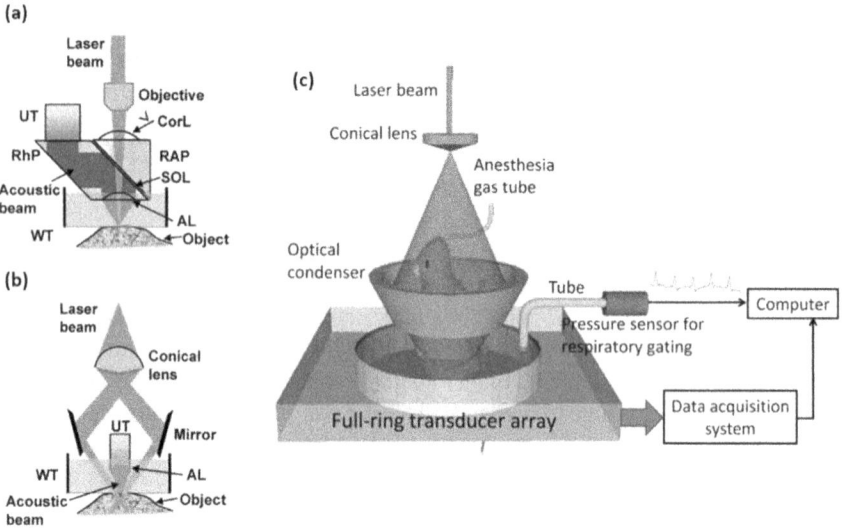

FIGURE 2.3 Experimental set-up of (a) OR-PAM; (b) AR-PAM; and (c) PACT.

optical focus to attain a high-resolution image while in AR-PAM, the laser beam is weakly focused and a focused transducer is used (Zhang et al., 2018).

Nonetheless, higher frequency and sensitivity detectors are needed in both PAM modalities to enable them for real-world clinical and pre-clinical applications. The lateral resolution and penetration depth that various PAI modalities can deliver, along with their main area of applications. The experimental setups of the PACT and PAM systems are shown in Figure 2.3.

2.4 CHALLENGES AND FUTURE PERSPECTIVE

From this review, one can appreciate the complexity of categorising photoacoustic imaging systems which are evolving into more robust equipment to facilitate clinical adoption. It can also be noted that the majority of the systems discussed here have been designed primarily at academic institutions, with only a few exceptions. These systems are therefore one-of-a-kind prototypes rather than final products. Since these systems were not designed for manufacturability and were developed to demonstrate feasibility with reasonable safety, they suffer from limited standardisation across the spectrum, making it almost impossible to compare data between the systems, posing a didactic challenge for the clinicians, not to mention the regulatory hurdles. Developments in system design to assume the form factor of clinical ultrasound scanners as suggested by recent advances is a step in the right direction to facilitate faster clinical integration filling this void. For photoacoustic imaging systems to be adopted widely, fast lasers that can operate at higher frame rates (hundreds or thousands of Hertz) similar to ultrasound for real-time image acquisition are important along with adequate safety monitoring systems that ensure safe laser-exposure levels for the patient and the provider.

Another key factor that impacts clinical adoption is the approval for marketing of the device for a specific clinical indication by regional regulatory bodies such as the FDA in the United States and CE Mark in the European Union. In light of the Affordable Care Act adopted in the United States recently, which imposes reimbursement penalties to healthcare facilities based on quality metrics, it has become increasingly complex for the medical device companies to bring new technologies for patient care as the healthcare sector is undergoing a major shift from a fee-for-service model to a value-based model, requiring companies to demonstrate value proposition clearly over existing standards of care at similar or lower adoption costs (Zhou et al., 2016). Therefore, it is important that the inventors consider such macroeconomic factors while developing commercial photoacoustic imaging systems in order to ensure a successful clinical translation. Several clinical trials on photoacoustic imaging that are currently underway (mostly first-in-human or phase I) focus on critical endpoints to demonstrate feasibility, safety and effectiveness. These trials, if successful, enable the need for subsequent larger phase II clinical trials that need to demonstrate value proposition to establish a robust reimbursement pathway which is a crucial factor for successful clinical adoption in addition to the safety and effectiveness data typically acquired for regulatory purposes. Formal health technology assessment programmes which are more common in Europe than in the United States (Chen et al., 2015) can be helpful during the early stages of photoacoustic imaging device development to anticipate any costs, challenges and pitfalls upfront and help mitigate the risks associated with business development and clinical adoption (Chen et al., 2017).

2.5 CONCLUSION

There is a growing interest in photoacoustic imaging among the key stakeholders including clinicians with several ongoing first-in-human clinical trials, as well as large medical device companies that are cautiously eager to acquire new technologies which are effective and carry minimal regulatory and reimbursement risks, allowing market penetration and adoption. Clinical applications discussed here highlight the potential of clinical photoacoustic imaging to complement ultrasound and other existing armaments to help combat cancer and hopefully ultimately ease its burden on the global healthcare system.

ACKNOWLEDGEMENTS

This work was supported by the Creative-Pioneering Researchers Program through Seoul National University (SNU), Korea.

REFERENCES

B. E. Treeby, E. Z. Zhang, and B. T. Cox, "Photoacoustic tomography in absorbing acoustic media using time reversal," *Inverse Probl.*, vol. 26, no. 11, p. 115003, 2010.
C. Kim, M. Jeon, and L. V. Wang, "Nonionizing photoacoustic cystography *in vivo*," *Opt. Lett.*, vol. 36, no. 18, pp. 3599–3601, 2011.

K. Sivasubramanian and M. Pramanik, "High frame rate photoacoustic imaging at 7000 frames per second using clinical ultrasound system," *Biomed. Opt. Express*, vol. 7, pp. 312–323, 2016.

M. Heijblom, *Breast imaging using light and sound*. Amsterdam: Nederlands Trial Register, 2011 [cited 2015 February 22]. Available from: http://www.trialregister.nl/trialreg/admin/rctview.asp?TC=2945.

P. Zhang, et al., "High-resolution deep functional imaging of the whole mouse brain by photoacoustic computed tomography in vivo," *J. Biophotonics*, vol. 11, no. 1, pp. 1–6, 2018.

S. L. Chen, L. J. Guo, and X. Wang, "All-optical photoacoustic microscopy," *Photoacoustics*, vol. 3, no. 4, pp. 143–150, 2015.

S. S. Gambhir, *Photoacoustic imaging (PAI) of the prostate: A clinical feasibility study.* Bethesda, MD: U.S. National Library of Medicine, 2012 [cited 2015 February 22]. Available from: https://clinicaltrials.gov/ct2/show/NCT01551576.

Y. Liu, L. Nie, and X. Chen, "Photoacoustic molecular imaging: From multiscale biomedical applications towards early-stage theranostics," *Trends Biotechnol.*, vol. 34, no. 5, p. 420, 2016.

Y. Petrova, Y. Y. Petrov, R. O. Esenaliev, D. J. Deyo, I. Cicenaite, and D. S. Prough, "Noninvasive monitoring of cerebral blood oxygenation in ovine superior sagittal sinus with novel multi-wavelength optoacoustic system," *Opt. Express*, vol. 17, no. 9, pp. 221–229, 2009.

Y. Zhou, J. Yao, and L. V. Wang, "Tutorial on photoacoustic tomography," *J. Biomed. Opt.*, vol. 21, no. 6, p. 061007, 2016.

Z. Chen, et al., "Non-invasive multimodal optical coherence and photoacoustic tomography for human skin imaging," *Sci. Rep.*, vol. 7, pp. 1–11, 2017.

3 Patient Empowerment of People with Rare Diseases

Neha Mehta and Archana Chaudhary

CONTENTS

3.1 INTRODUCTION TO PATIENT EMPOWERMENT

Patient empowerment is a two-fold process that allows the patient to control their health and actions wherein the patients have their health-related data and they share it with their caregivers. This helps the patients with their accurate and real-time diagnoses. Patient empowerment is the informed mode of control of one's own health through the self mode and the collective mode. Patient empowerment is a way of motivating the patients so that they know the benefits of treatement [1]. The patients assume responsibility for their own health. According to a statement by the WHO in 1978, the people have the right and the duty to get involved both individually and collectively in the planning and implementation of healthcare. According to the Council of the European Union, the involvement of the patients is declared as the common operating principle. Thus, the empowerment of the patient may be defined as a process that occurs at both the individual level and the collective level

DOI: 10.1201/9781003132110-3

within the medical context and without. Patient empowerment, in turn, produces long-term solutions for disease management [2]. The patient tends to act as an active partner who can be a rational self-manager and real-time decision-maker regarding their health and also ensures the disease effects minimise. In addition, the patients suffering from chronic diseases also reduce the burden of the health sector. Thus, many resources have shifted from a disease-oriented approach to a patient-oriented approach. But the field of patient empowerment is very heterogeneous and multi-dimensional. The influence of the main keyword, that is, power, has revealed the ability of the patients with regard to what they need. Patient empowerment is a field of both practical and theory domains with the aspect of power and powerlessness. It enhances the personal, community-based and interpersonal power of improving a condition. It also includes the visibility of sub-processes like awareness, accepting self-responsibility, developing positive attitudes, improving self-efficacy and much more. However, in the context of chronic diseases, there is an involvement of certain goals in disease management that includes psychologically treating patients through responding, counselling, advising and educating towards the building up of a positive attitude, confidence and self-perception. According to P. Freire [3], patient empowerment has a direct link with the process of education intervention by shifting the patients to act autonomously and to think critically. Patient empowerment is gaining prominence these days due to its equitable and more collaborative way of health delivery along with cost-effectiveness.

3.1.1 HISTORY AND CONCEPT

The historical overview of empowerment is similar in essence to the principles of increasing the ability of groups and individuals to ensure their wellbeing and their decision-making rights. P. Freire in 1960 has given an important and influential concept about "popular education" which later came to be part of development practices in 1970 in the entirety of Latin America. However, it came into effect in the 1980s when empowerment had come to be seen in most areas through social transformation and collectively claiming rights. A renowned example related to health was noted in 1983 during the empowerment drive for the people who were living with acquired immunodeficiency syndrome. From that context [3], empowerment has got an increase in its interventions and research for the groups who are experiencing marginalisation. According to Gibson, empowerment may be easily understood as the absence of hopelessness, powerlessness, victimisation, alienation, oppression and other negative feelings that have the least control of one's own life and an increase in dependency [4]. The World Bank also defines empowerment as the process of increasing the capacity of persons and groups in order to make their choice and also to transform their choices into the desired actions. This in turn is a build-up of the assets that increase organisational efficiency.

However, in the 20th century, patient empowerment has received prominence as a method to get away from paternalism and use more collaborative models towards healthcare delivery. Empowerment results in the activation of patients on the one end and thus the rejection of passivity on the other. It helps the patients in assuming their duty towards self-care. EMPATHiE, an EU-funded project for the management of patients suffering from chronic diseases, has highlighted that an empowered patient controls the management of the condition of their life. Thus, patient empowerment can be seen as the dynamic approach to changing multiple strategies according to the way in which one co-operates and manages in order to enter everyday life by developing self-confidence towards physical, social and emotional aspects of life. The process of patient empowerment is a process that occurs at both individual (micro) level and collective (macro) level, both in terms of health-based quality and social services. The key components of patient empowerment include:

1. Understanding the patient
2. Acquisition of the patient's knowledge
3. The skills of the patient
4. A facilitating environment

The calculation of the impact of difficulties, formal barriers and informal barriers towards relations (personal and between communities) is important for people with rare diseases. According to the research, the group of people with their diseases may be collectively dealt with through collaborative treatment instead of independent treatment towards their empowerment and social recognition. However, the coordination between the patients, physicians and caregivers is the key component to develop self-empowerment among the people where self-care has prime importance.

Along with having control of one's health, there are five important qualities that are identified as the keys to patient empowerment as mentioned below:

1. Literacy and education
2. Expertise in dealing
3. Interactive decision-making
4. Experience sharing
5. Self-engagement

Being a literate, educated and informed person towards one's own health is one of the important resources of empowerment. The improvement in health literacy evenly improves the cost as well as the contribution of the healthcare system. According to the WHO, when the patient's literacy level is limited, it also has a negative impact on the patient's health, thus it is required that the patient should get involved in the interaction process of exchange of health-related information. Also, the patients should know about trustworthy and reliable sources of information.

3.2 MODERATORS AND INTERVENTIONS

The moderators of empowerment are the variables that influence the outcome of any desired functionality. In patient empowerment, the functionality of shared decisions for any patient is applicable if more than one specialist doctor is involved in the diagnosis and treatment of the patient. In that case, the characteristics of the healthcare provider, his training values, personal experiences and many more are the moderators which can cause implications for patient empowerment. Similarly, at the patient level, the moderators are his social values, disease severity and moral values. There is always a dual relationship between patient behaviour and patient capacities. The patient capacity is always expected to be improved through empowerment and enhancing health literacy.

Similarly, the moderators existing at the level of the healthcare system include legislatory factors, political contexts, priority setting and many more.

However, while implementing patient empowerment in a healthcare organisation, the consideration of various factors necessitates the development of impacts through moderators due to which the major interventions at both the patient level and the healthcare level are identified. Thus, there always exists the effects of moderators on the patient values and the healthcare providers' professional goals. Thus, the varieties of interventions are faced at the promoting levels of patient empowerment. Studies have also found that the implementation of interventions depending upon behaviour, health and patient satisfaction has given a positive effect on health. The interventions for promoting patient care along with clinical consultations are found more effective. According to many studies, patient-empowering interventions are classified under two broad categories:

1. Individual-focused interventions
2. Group-focused interventions

There are several further techniques under these two; for 1) individual-focused interventions, the individual patient deals with various procedures in order to make him a focused empowered patient. That may be with the help of patient-centred interview, true motivational counselling and special coaching. The shared decision method, according to the authors [5], describes the shared decision as a three-step technique defined under intervention for promoting patient empowerment. The process of shared decision is a three-step process to be done by healthcare providers through the introduction of all the available choices of care to the patient, as a first step. In the second step, the decision-supporting tools are used for describing all the possible options to the patient. In the third step, the patients are helped to explore all the preferences and thus make a suitable decision. Another intervention class is a group-focused intervention in which the uniform groups of patients are created and the empowering techniques are implemented. The various techniques of this category include expert interaction, self-management skills, personalised care and planning, disease-based education, etc. Researchers [6] have investigated personalised interventions and have informed that culturally specific interventions are essential to be involved in the patient's treatment. According to the research, patient empowerment and activation are part of a cyclic process, where patient engagement is referred to as a "blockbuster drug" [7]. According to ACA, the Affordable Care Act, the treatment of the patient includes the provisions to encourage the healthcare providers to engage "oneself", with the patients as proactive participants for maintaining their health and effectiveness in their self-management of chronic diseases. In contrast, less engagement of patients towards prevention and continuing wellness is one of the factors that are reported for disease severity, especially among minorities.

PAE, or the personalised activation and empowerment of a patient, is referred to as a combination of two mutually dependent tasks, i.e. patient activation and patient empowerment. The patient activation is concerned with self-knowledge and skills to manage one's health. However, patient empowerment is the involvement of one's efficacy and self-capacity in order to make decisions. Patient empowerment is the concept that reflects more determination and confidence for making autonomous decisions. Ultimately it can also be marked that the combination of both empowerment and activation enhances the confidence and knowledge of the patient towards their health, treatment and healthcare through healthcare providers and even with policy interventions. However, in the care of patients with rare diseases, the task of patient empowerment plays an even greater role. According to the research, it has been reported that patients with rare diseases often share the same set of experiences, irrespective of the fact that each disease has its own set of symptoms and characteristics. The challenges being faced by rare disease patients include low prevalence, less treatment, limited knowledge, restricted lifestyle, fatigue, depression, anxiety, limited participation in society and many more. In addition to this, a hidden fact is also real about their disrespect and a disregard for them from the research community and policy makers [8]. This class requires action-oriented empowerment in order to eradicate the formal and informal barriers. Thus, the medical community is suggested to identify the people with rare diseases and collectively address them towards joint actions for their strengthening. Some of the common practices in search of community towards their empowerment include improvement of access towards knowledge, enhancement in social support, reducing social exclusion, improving lifestyle and much more. Such practices are needed to be carried out at both the individual level and the society level. Web-based activities may also play an eminent role in this empowerment by introducing the joint community online, between cross-border people. Similarly, the introduction of helplines and support services give the essential lacking information to search persons.

3.3 ROLE OF ICT IN PATIENT EMPOWERMENT

In order to improve patient knowledge and information, access to such tools is required, so that health literacy gets improved and the patient must come under the category of an informed patient. The knowledge about their health and their diseases should be given to the patients, as their fundamental right. For the further approach, the patient should know about the conditions and options to control their disease. Thus, for the control of their health data and knowledge, the patient needs an approach towards the technology, which often helps them to track their health data and download it according to their choice. Similarly, the physicians also need scalable tools that help to maintain autonomy about patient records and improvement. The feature of shared decision-making is also one of the important tools which engage the patient along with their physicians for motivation and further development. Many researchers have accomplished their work in this particular field and have reported the implementation of technology to be the transforming role-player in patient empowerment.

Patient engagement tools are one of the best options catering in this category, which aim to activate the patients for their own benefit and also to streamline the experience of the patients. According to a research study published in the *Journal of Medical Internet Research*, adolescent patients are on the cusp of disease management. Thus, m-Health applications are beneficial aids for them. Along with m-Health applications, self-management support is also an inspiration for the patients between their medical visits. The m-Health applications can be easily installed on smartphones, which enables them to be fitness trackers. Just like diet tracking, counters and fitness tracking are the prominently used applications that are even commonly being used by every individual as a part of remote monitoring.

The special features of ICT being implemented in m-Health are also being widely used for accomplishing telemedicine and remote patient monitoring. The wearable devices like Fitbits and Apple watches are tools to manage the overall wellness of patients. The ICT, which is involved in m-Health, has allowed connectivity between patients and providers even in disparate locations, along with the monitoring of the patients outside the clinic. However, there may be many challenges faced by the patients and the providers in the way they perceive the technology and the way they interact with m-Health applications. But m-Health has given opportune time for engagement and preventive care.

The use of ICT has proved to be more beneficial for the task of patient engagement by introducing empowerment-based ICT applications in which the patient gets an opportunity to see their physical information—also in more than just emergency conditions—which gives motivation and more power to control their health in all aspects.

3.3.1 Barriers in Operability

Sometimes, the limited operability of internet or broadband access in rural sites and the improper working of the applications have become the most prominent barriers in patient empowerment using m-Health. The other hidden reasons, which are acting as the silent barriers, include more time consumption in entering the data, the related hidden costs, the confusing nature of the application for less literate people, language issues and apprehension towards data sharing. The consumers are also facing issues with the interfaces of the apps in terms of accuracy, while calculation of parameters and data security are also issues.

3.4 MEASURING PATIENT EMPOWERMENT

The implementation of patient empowerment has been in a range of wide contexts. The expression of patient empowerment is one of the primarily adopted bases for approaches towards patient health. Due to its wide consensus of importance and largely accepted multidimensional nature, a large variety of empowerment parameters are coming into action. According to P. Freire's philosophy, empowerment is one of the better solutions towards oppression and inequality faced by the patients. Empowerment is always viewed as a characteristic towards community transformation instead of that of any single individual. According to the research, certain dimensions of patient empowerment have been found. They are:

1. Participation in shared decisions
2. Knowledge acquisition
3. Positive attitude towards health
4. Control over health
5. Capacity building

While measuring patient empowerment, the empowerment can be process-oriented or outcome-oriented. The attributes responsible for process-oriented empowerment include obeying the patient's choice, communication between the patient and the healthcare practitioners, shared or autonomous decision-making and thus completing a successful treatment. However, outcome-oriented empowerment is the one where if increased levels of a patient's motivation, confidence and health improvement are attained, then successful patient empowerment on the basis of outcome is said to be attained.

Thus, in empowerment, an enabling process is developed in which the healthcare professionals collaborate along with the patients and a system for helping them to acquire a resource of the best knowledge with balanced and informed decisions. Another major aspect is called patient enablement. Patient enablement is conceptually an indicator of self-efficacy and is also associated with behaviours like self-care and treatment adherence. Patient enablement often describes the clinical encounter towards the patient's ability to understand the illness. Along with the encouragement of the patient in realising self-autonomy, there are four known levels of patient empowerment: level 1: the patient acts more paternalistic; level 2: the patient has a demanding nature; level 3: informed consent; and level 4: informed decision, as there is always an expectation for growing updates between patient knowledge and patient decision-making. Figure 3.1 shows these parameters with the levels of patient empowerment.

Along with this, the valid reasons for measuring patient empowerment include:

1. Ethical reasons
2. Understanding the development of services
3. System enforcement
4. Maintaining clinical governance or auditing reasons

The parameters that are needed to be measured for the level of empowerment are:

1. Patient's view about his/her care
2. Evaluation of healthcare procedure by a higher number of users
3. Level of patient involvement in self-care
4. Level of patient satisfaction

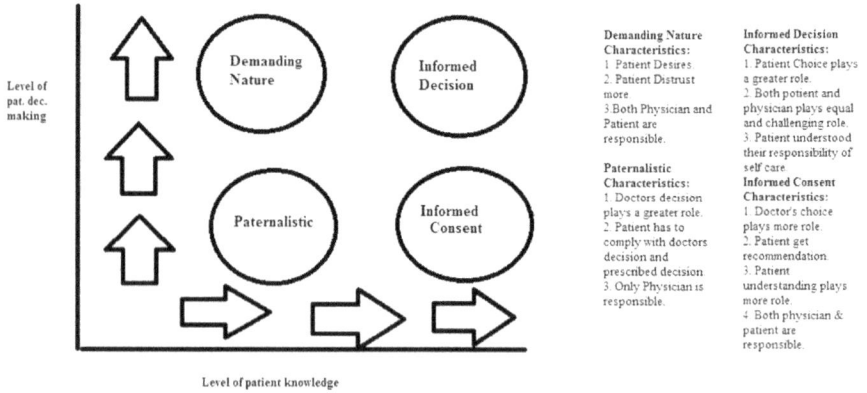

Level of
pat. dec.
making

Demanding
Nature

Informed
Decision

Paternalistic

Informed
Consent

Level of patient knowledge

**Demanding Nature
Characteristics:**
1. Patient Desires
2. Patient Distrust
more
3. Both Physician and
Patient are
responsible.

**Paternalistic
Characteristics:**
1. Doctors decision
plays a greater role.
2. Patient has to
comply with doctors
decision and
prescribed decision
3. Only Physician is
responsible.

**Informed Decision
Characteristics:**
1. Patient Choice plays
a greater role.
2. Both patient and
physician plays equal
and challenging role.
3. Patient understood
their responsibility of
self care.

**Informed Consent
Characteristics:**
1. Doctor's choice
plays more role.
2. Patient get
recommendation.
3. Patient
understanding plays
more role.
4. Both physician &
patient are
responsible.

FIGURE 3.1   Different levels of patient empowerment.

5. Level of patient confidence
6. Level of enhancement in the patient's trust for his doctor and/or caretaker

The parameters that are needed to be measured for checking the patient's view about the quality of healthcare include:

1. Preferences
2. Evaluations
3. Reports

Preferences, along with priorities are often used in the context of empowerment that are used to refer the patient's views and ideas about their clinical treatment and the Healthcare system. However, the priorities describe the preferences of the volume of persons. The strategies used to measure preferences are: (1) qualitative methods and (2) quantitative methods.

In the qualitative methods, the system uses different techniques to conduct person-to-person interviews. However, the quantitative method includes the different processes of conducting surveys or consensus methods. The strategies of measuring evaluations include quantitative methods like a set of questionnairse, getting the questionnaires filled in by patients and their caretakers. The qualitative method for measuring the evaluation includes the analysis of quantitative surveys and thus measuring the reliability of such surveys. Reports are the strategies of reporting the objective observations about the healthcare system and the related services, which may be used for improving the quality and standard of the system.

Factors influencing the responsive rate of the patients include: (a) motivation factor, (b) user-friendly questionnaire, (c) monetary incentives, (d) administering the benefits of filling the questionnaires, (e) level of satisfaction of the patients, (f) services of the healthcare system, (g) literacy level of the patients and (h) frequency of visiting the healthcare institution.

3.5 GAP BETWEEN SOCIAL CARE AND HEALTHCARE OF RARE DISEASES

A gap between social care and healthcare needs to be bridged for persons with rare diseases; this is quite an urgent need to be filled. The persons with rare diseases often feel less support from healthcare as well as social care. However, it is not only a requirement but also important to offer to such people quality of life, autonomy and support for the realisation of fundamental rights. Due to their special needs which are socially unmet, and the complex nature of the disease, such people must be given special attention. Along with this, the policy makers have also initialised an important policy process towards an approach for rare diseases involving the provision of holistic care.

There are different definitions of rare diseases given by different countries, according to their respective populations and healthcare systems. According to the WHO, rare diseases are debilitating disorders prevailing in ≤ 1 in 1,000 of the population. According to the US, a rare disease affects 6.4 in 10,000 people [9]. However, the EU defines it as a life-threatening condition affecting not more than 5 out of 10,000 persons. However, according to the NGO committee for rare diseases, established under CoNGO, person with rare diseases face many challenges such as accessibility to proper treatment, healthcare services, infrastructure and understandable information about self-care. They have also reported the human rights which need to be addressed including the right to health, quality of life and right to life for the persons affected by rare diseases.

3.6 INDICATORS OF PATIENT EMPOWERMENT

On the basis of patient capacities, states and available resources, the following indicators assure patient empowerment.

1. Skills and attitudes towards one's own health
2. Self-efficacy
3. Evaluating sense and coherence
4. Participation in shared decisions
5. Playing an active role in health consultations
6. Ability to make informed and shared decisions
7. Using the internet to increase health information

3.7 OUTCOMES AND IMPACT OF PATIENT EMPOWERMENT ON THE ENTIRE HEALTH SYSTEM

The nature of rare diseases may be chronic, genetic or life-threatening, and the diagnosis has always been a challenge for physicians and patients due to continuously increasing population and variation in the disease behaviour. The adequacy of biomarkers and the screening protocols leads to non-diagnosis for many rare diseases. For most healthcare organisations, patient treatment is said to be effective and improved on the basis of patient satisfaction seen at the healthcare centre. Sometimes the health data may be complex and also the access to health tools is difficult to be navigated. Thus, promoting interoperability and better communication has produced effective health outcomes. The implementation of the experience which is received from the interoperable healthcare legislation and from stack story examples (like HIPAA) has led to a successful improvement in the health outcomes. In Coleman et al. [10], the researchers have produced that in many of the developing countries, and the beginning of patient empowerment got started in the 1950s for the people living with chronic diseases. Starting from the patient assertions, the second approach was epistemological, that the patient judges their experience and knowledge, and the third was about the political claim, where the patients get involved in their health decisions. These claims had eventually produced an acknowledgement of empowered health outcomes. The patients suffering from rare diseases along with their caring organisations are the most empowered clusters of the empowered health sector. The researchers have also produced the idea for an emerging expert patient where the expert patient is a patient who emerges as a reflexive consumer for making active decisions.

The outcomes and impacts of patient empowerment may be listed as:

1. Patients' adaptation towards their illness
2. Comfortability for their quality of life
3. Satisfaction about treatment
4. Tracking the disease
5. Improvement in the clinical health status

3.8　ROLE OF PATIENT PORTALS

Patient portals are the special and secured websites prepared for the patients in order to maintain the regular practices of the healthcare provider. It is meant to deliver the multiple numbers of functions that are linked with the electronic health record. The patient portals involve protected medical information, pathology reports and appointment schedules along with secure message delivery. The patient portals also tend to offer various programmes for the self-management of the patients. It offers a continuous approach towards patient adherence, patient empowerment, patient caretaker communication and patient satisfaction. The way of engaging the patients towards their healthcare delivery always adds to the potential for improving the health outcomes of the patients and their level of satisfaction. The patients are engaged by enabling them to access their electronic medical records (EMR). The patient portals serve as a kind of e-visit, just like a house call in which the patient is not required to wait for the official hours, but they can access their data, summaries, test reports and even make appointments anytime. This is even more supported with a list of specialists available and all the types of treatments available. However, the providers can also see and manage the disease history of the patients along with the gentle advice that has been given earlier.

3.8.1 Dimensions of Patient Portals

On the basis of different applications of patient portals in healthcare, they are supposed to accomplish many of the tedious and time-taking tasks in an easier way. Thus, the different dimensions of patient portals in the healthcare sector are shown in Figure 3.2.

In support of the premise, patient portals are serving as complex interventions that have multiple pathways through different domains in order to generate different outcomes. The patient portals have served as a regular and frequently used mechanism for patients' insight into their continuity of care. The different domains of patient portals have allowed the patients insight into information, continuity of care and more convenience.

- *Design*: The design dimension includes the designing of the portal including its features, content and interfaces.
- *Organisation*: The organisation includes the decision basis, action culture of the healthcare organisation and the organisational consideration towards the implementation of a patient portal.
- *Usage*: The usage includes helping the staff and patients to be more equipped with the training and necessary skills for making effective use of patient portals.
- *Facilitators*: The facilitators are meant to enable the users to understand the functionalities and make them more comfortable by motivating them to use patient portals.
- *Barriers*: The barriers may be infrastructural or technical and may hinder the usage of patient portals for both patients and practitioners.
- *Output and benefits*: Active engagement is always associated with the benefits and better outcomes for portal users that may be in terms of time-saving, comfortability, relaxing or even early disease indication.

However, the complexity of these dimensions needs a special emphasis and a necessity of further research that can disentangle them in order to provide the related outcomes.

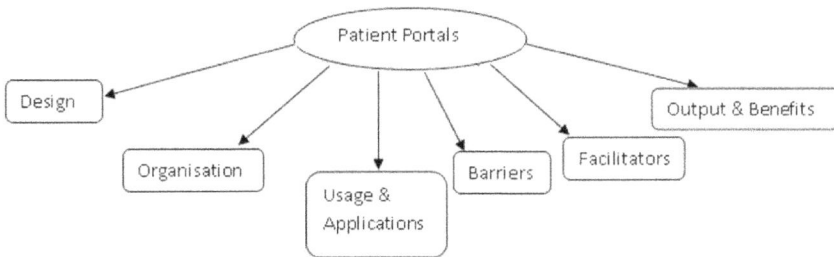

FIGURE 3.2 Dimensions of patient portals.

3.8.2 SPECIALISED SERVICES

The specialised services are the well-known services that are reported as instrumental to the empowerment of persons with rare diseases, along with their wellbeing and health. Recently, EURORDIS (European Committee of Experts for Rare Diseases) has become the upcoming leader in their work for specialised services in Europe. The services are:

A. Delivering respite care services
B. Development of resource centres
C. Promoting adapted housing
D. Organising therapeutic recreation programmes

Similarly, the NPTRD (National Policy for Treatment of Rare Diseases) was designed by the Ministry of Health and Family Welfare, Government of India, in the year 2017. According to the reports, the field of rare diseases is heterogeneous in nature and complex as well. As per the researchers, this field has a constantly changing landscape, in which new conditions and diseases are constantly arising.

3.9 EVERMORE, DEALING WITH THE RD COMMUNITIES

3.9.1 OUTCOME MEASUREMENT

Patients and their caregivers are substituted as the advocates for persons with rare diseases (RD), due to their role in creating awareness and also in describing the daily progress and manifestations of the diseases and the ongoing treatment. The outcome measurement and the RD research of the patient depend on the lab measurements, treatment and observations, imaging data, genomic data, etc. However, the big challenge for their diagnosis is the reporting through EHRs and the existing clinical information systems. The major resources for RDs include OMIM, GARD, MedGen and Orphanet. In most cases, the patient presentations are so heterogeneous that they may not exactly match the symptoms of earlier experienced diseases.

The RD patient outcome depends on the following:

1. The successful demonstration of the clinical effectiveness.
2. Measurement of the factors that affect the patients.
3. The successful understanding of the treatment and related clinical decisions.
4. Effective demonstration of the clinical outcomes.
5. Interpretation of disease endpoints.
6. Improved drug efficacy.

However, the methods which are used in qualitative research are involved in the outcome measurement as shown in Figure 3.3.

An alignment of the rare diseases is dependent on the overall patient outcome that may be calculated on the basis of the integration of the impacts of the different domains. Investigational research is always known as a step ahead towards multiple endpoints.

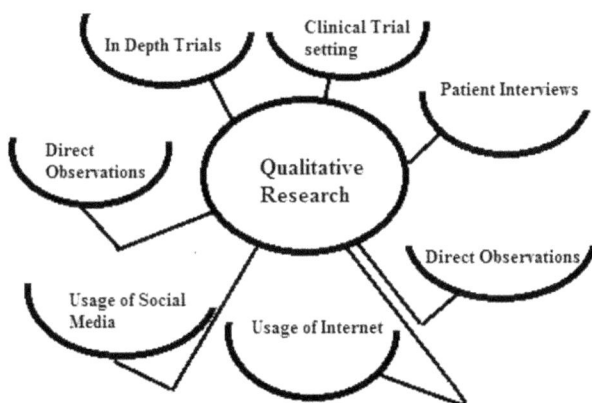

FIGURE 3.3 Outcomes of qualitative research.

3.9.2 TOWARDS RD CLINICAL RESEARCH (RDCR)

RD registries are the backbone of clinical research in this domain and are crucial for management and increasing patient care, health planning and quality of life outcomes. The registries are classified as:

a. Population-based RDCR
b. Hospital-based RDCR

However, in both of the RDCR methods, the patient and the related conditions are the primary sources of information. But there is a continuous transformation in the physician data according to the regular capturing of experienced data. These are referred to as the primary sources of data and EHR are the secondary sources of data. The managed and updated registries are the methods that are adapted to collect the data and identify the phenotypes. In this way, the registries accomplish the patient's needs and also their priorities.

In order to deal with the RD (rare disease) communities, the following important points have crucial values in disease management and treatment:

- The assurance that they are an active role player and ensuring them about effective engagement at all levels of decision making.
- Involvement of patients in steering committees, overseeing the implementations.
- Recognition of the roles of patients and the representatives in the healthcare centres.
- Integration of the patients according to clinical trial protocol design along with the patient outcomes.
- Promoting their training for education and capacity-building initiatives.
- Supporting environment for their empowerment initiatives even through public money.

- Guaranteed approval and progress for the rare disease policies by maintaining volatility in the political background.
- Reinforcement of the care managers as role players for addressing the range of needs of rare disease patients and also navigating the environmental conditions.
- Adapting for social services in order to cater to the RD patients' needs and for promoting their inclusion in the national social policies, thus allowing for their integration in societies, workplaces and living communities.

REFERENCES

1. De Santis, M., et al., "Patient empowerment of people living with rare diseases. Its contribution to sustainable and resilient healthcare systems", *Annali dell'Istituto superiore di sanita*, 2019, Vol. 55, No. 3, 283–291.
2. Vainauskien, V., and Vaitkien, R., "Enablers of patient knowledge empowerment for self-management of chronic disease: An integrative review", *International Journal of Environmental Research and Public Health*, 2021,Vol. 18, 2247.
3. Anderson, R. M., and Funnell, M. M., "Patient empowerment: Myths and misconceptions", *Patient Education and Counseling*, 2010, Vol. 79, 277–282.
4. Gibson, C. H., "A concept analysis of empowerment", *Journal of Advanced Nursing*, 1991, Vol. 16, No. 3, 354–361.
5. Bravo, P., et al., "Conceptualising patient empowerment: A mixed methods study", *BMC Health Services Research*, 2015, Vol. 15, 252.
6. Chen, J., et al., "Personalized strategies to activate and empower patients in health care and reduce health disparities", *Health Education & Behavior*, 2016, Vol. 43, No. 1, 25–34.
7. Kish, I., "The blockbuster drug of the century: An engaged patient", 2014. Available at: http://www.hl7standards.com/blog/2012/08/28/drug-of-the-century/.
8. Elwyn, G., et al., "Shared decision making: A model for clinical practice", *Journal of General Internal Medicine*, 2012, Vol. 27, 1361–1367.
9. Nagaraja, S., et al., "A comparative study of orphan drugs in US, EU & India", 2018. Available at: http://pharmabiz.com/NewsDetails.aspx?aid=108801&sid=21#:~:text=Initially%20a%20guideline%20(Orphan%20Drug,disease%20as%20a%20life%2Dthreatening
10. Coleman, K., et al., "Evidence on the chronic care model in the new millennium", *Health Affairs*, 2009, Vol. 28, 75–85.

4 A Systematic Approach to Agricultural Drones Using a Machine Learning Model

S. Arunmozhiselvi, T. Ananth Kumar,
P. Manju Bala, S. Usharani and G. Glorindal

CONTENTS

DOI: 10.1201/9781003132110-4

4.1   INTRODUCTION

The global economy is critically dependent on agriculture. More people mean a greater demand for food, which may stress the agricultural systems. Precision-based agriculture, which has emerged as a new scientific field using less resource-intensive techniques to increase productivity while controlling environmental impact, is a combination of data-intensive techniques and other scientific fields. Adhering to accurate and frequent operational conditions (i.e. crop and soil conditions) allows for faster and more efficient decision-making.

This powerful combination of new data technologies and efficient production machines has given us brand new prospects to unpick and quantify the study methods. Every year, ML is used in new scientific fields, for example, bioinformatics, weather prediction and agriculture and climate research, in addition to its traditional roles in biological, medical and technological fields. Agriculture is the Indian economy's backbone. Every day in agriculture, many new technologies are introduced, which can be costly and require high electricity consumption. Farmers face every obstacle in agriculture.

4.1.1   Machine Learning

Machine learning, a sub-class of artificial intelligence, is an approach to artificial intelligence that leverages algorithms that help the system learn from the training it has already undergone. An example of this would be the kind of data given as input to the system and the pattern it finds in that data, which it then uses to provide an output. With time, the system grows smarter and wiser on its own. It uses a statistical learning algorithm that learns and improves automatically without the need for human assistance. This machine learning and UAV-blending make more precise, more accurate and more efficient image classification as well as feasible object detection.

4.1.2   Supervised Learning

The term "supervised learning" is more specifically applied to training, where the teacher assists and directs students in doing the assignments. For machine learning purposes, we have to allow the machine to see or instruct itself with correct information using proper labels. This means that data has already been tagged with the answer. Then, the supervised learning algorithm is given a set of data and works through this set of training examples to find a correct outcome [1].

For example, if a basket full of various fruits is given, as shown in Figure 4.1, consider the following situation: first, expand the machine's training with new foods one by one until the patterns have been learned. Red will be chosen for anything that is both rounded and convex. Now suppose you have put a new fruit into the basket, such as a banana, as shown in Figure 4.2. If you want to know which one, then place it in the expansion chamber and leave the others alone and ask. This new data has already been incorporated into the learning algorithm. Thus, it will utilise all previous data more effectively. A banana can be referred to as lotus-leaf black or expanded into a comprehensive approach like lotus-yellow before being identified as an actual banana. The algorithm can then perform more complex tasks involving fruits (simple or complex tasks that the machine has learned in training) by doing so (new fruit) [2].

The supervised learning technique has been divided into two heuristics: simple classification and complex regression technique. When you ask a question about "disease" or "colour," the category "red" or "blue" or "not diseased" is expanded to "is red, diseased, or is diseased". When the output variable is "money" rather than

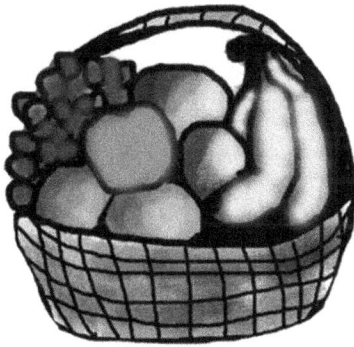

FIGURE 4.1   Fruit basket.

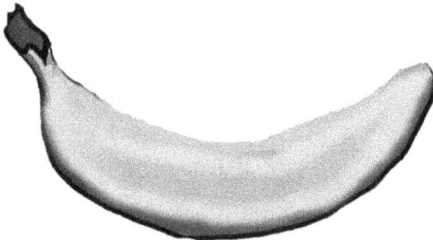

FIGURE 4.2   Classified object by trained machine.

numeric, a stable relationship is a difficulty that has developed between the forecast and the result variable. Unsupervised learning is about data labelled as "Yes" or "No". Some data tagged with the correct answer in this example is being used in other sentences. The supervised method of training a machine learning model is used to gather data and predict previous experiences. Supervised machine learning narrows the goals by optimising the performance criteria. A specific kind of learning algorithm, supervised learning, helps to deal with a wide range of different kinds of real-world issues [3].

4.1.3 UNSUPERVISED LEARNING

Unsupervised learning is the technique where the algorithm is given no intervention by humans, free to perform without direct supervision. The machines identify patterns, find relationships that have been unknown previously, cluster information according to their characteristics and unearth novel information. More education is better than training, and there are no bad habits to break because there is no master. The computer does this without assistance. Suppose an image consists of both dogs and cats, which it has never seen. The machine does not know about the specific characteristics of dogs and cats, which prevents them from being classified as "dogs and cats". To recap, the above-mentioned picture can be classified according to similarities, patterns and differences, e.g. it is pretty simple to categorise this picture into two separate parts. Consider the example shown in Figure 4.3, if the first may contain all pictures of dogs, and the second part may contain all pictures of cats, it can be said that the first contains all images of dogs, and the second part contains all images of cats. No training data or examples, in this case, are received, which means there was no prior knowledge to expand on. It enables the model to do its work and discover patterns and information that would not have been discovered without it. Data that is not labelled is mainly dealt with in this document [2].

4.1.4 MACHINE LEARNING TERMINOLOGIES

Machine learning follows a training process to learn from training data to perform a given task. A single instance will feature various characteristics and be referred to as an example. The feature may be a number in the form of a cardinal or ordinal number, such as "one" or "zero". Determining the model's accuracy in a particular

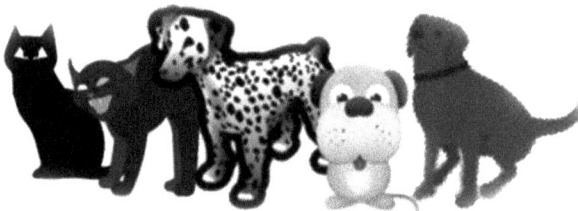

FIGURE 4.3 Example diagram for unsupervised learning.

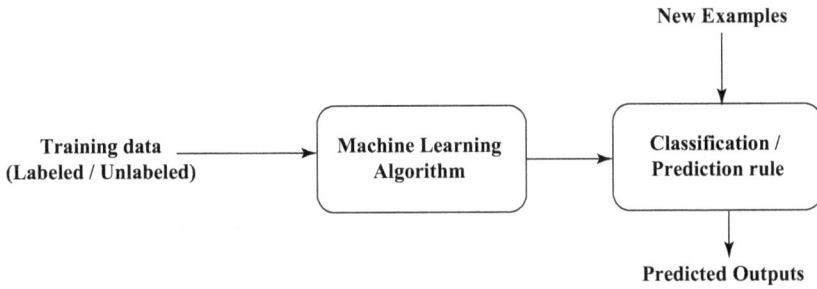

FIGURE 4.4   Procedure of a machine learning approach.

task entails evaluating the model's performance on that task and tracking how the model's performance improves with training. ML models and algorithms are extensively used in order to estimate their performance. Once the trained model is completed, it can predict, classify or cluster new testing data using the newly acquired training. The machine learning model is given in Figure 4.4. Unsupervised learning describes the majority of ML problems [2].

4.1.5   LEARNING TASKS IN MACHINE LEARNING

In learning, tasks are subdivided into supervised and unsupervised learning, depending on whether the signal input given to the training model is a learning signal. The machine receives several examples to use in comparison to the corresponding input. An example of a system that incorporates the dynamic environment in which inputs are only partially available links different training cycles with feedback back to training interventions in a dynamic environment (reinforcement learning). Once the procured expertise (trained model) predicts unknown output results (labels) for the test data, supervised settings produce good results. Unsupervised learning, even so, is a scenario where the training and test data are un-labelled. The learner looks for hidden patterns within the input data in order to improve understanding.

4.1.6   ANALYSIS OF LEARNING

According to machine learning (ML), the operation of dimensionality reduction (DR) is used in both supervised and unsupervised learning algorithms. The processing objective is to generate a concise and low-level representation of a set of data while retaining as much information as possible while keeping the dataset. The scientists would first use a classification or regression model to determine dimensions before applying dimensionality to ensure that the results do not contain dimensional data. Many of the most popular machine learning algorithms have numerous drawbacks and should therefore be avoided. The principal component analysis involves running regressions on all available data to find the component with the most significant magnitude, as well as linear discriminant analysis.

4.1.7 LEARNING MODELS

There is a variety of learning models from which one can choose, but we present just the ones that have been used in these studies.

4.1.7.1 Regression

Regression follows a supervised learning model that attempts to deliver predictions for a particular output variable, such as revenue, by deriving it from fixed and identifiable input variables. Another method that can be employed is ordinary least squares regression, which has more complex mathematical algorithms.

4.1.7.2 Clustering

Clustering is a common technique for applying unsupervised learning models, which are frequently employed to predict the natural association of data (clusters) with their properties and behaviour. For many years, three effective techniques have been used and include the K-means clustering method, the hierarchical clustering method and the expectation-maximisation method.

4.1.7.3 Bayesian Models

There are many families of probabilistic graphical models called Bayesian models (BMs). In this family, the analysis is done to help one to apply Bayesian inference. The use of the classification methodology was originally supervised learning variety and is particularly adept at classifying or regressing problems. Numerous techniques are mentioned in the literature, including naive Bayes, Gaussian naive Bayes, multinomial naive Bayes, Bayesian networks, Gaussian mixtures and Bayesian belief networks.

4.1.7.4 Instance-Based Models

Instance-based models (IBMs) use memory-based learning methods. They examine new examples to determine how they relate to already-seen instances in the training database. In contrast to those which maintain abstractions and try to formulate classifications or regression predictions, they draw their classifications and regression predictions from the actual data they have at hand. Their models have a significant disadvantage: the intricacy of their models begins to grow with new data. This learning algorithm class can be subdivided into the most frequently used ones, including a k-nearest neighbour, locally weighted learning and learning vector quantisation.

4.1.7.5 Ensemble Learning

Ensemble learning is a method for appropriately generating and combining various brands such as classification models to solve a particular computational intelligence problem. Ensemble learning is mostly used to help classify, predict, and approximate functions. These are used in statistical data and machine learning to achieve higher accuracy than all other constituent learning algorithms.

4.1.7.6 Decision Trees

The architecture of decision trees is a tree-like structure, as are their respective classification and regression models. As each subset is broken down, decision trees (DT) will keep track of each population, allowing for the development of a tree graph that visualises the structure of the population. Each branch on the tree represents a comparison result on a selected feature in each node, whereas each branch serves as an input for other nodes. As the path continues to the leaf, the node is defined as the final decision or prediction made as a result of the process originating from the root (expressed as a classification rule). There are several types of learning algorithms employed in this category. One of the most commonly used algorithms is a classification and regression tree, also known as the chi-square automatic interaction detector.

4.1.7.7 Models Behind

While reading about the future can be exciting, it is essential to consider the technologies that make it possible. It is, for instance, an established collection of models and algorithms that collect specific data and use them to deliver specific results. So far, machine learning and distribution methods in agriculture have been uneven. When machine learning is used in crop management processes, such as irrigation management, crop-growth scheduling, and crop residue management, that is considered the most prominent application. According to the literature review, the most popular agricultural models are ANNs and DL, while SVMs follow at a reasonably distant third. The application of ANNs to neural networks, which includes pattern generation, cognition, learning and decision making, is modelled on the biological implementation of ANNs. These models are utilised in weed, disease or attribute detection. Deep learning artificial neural networks have broadened the applications for ANNs in all fields, including agriculture. The yield and quality of crops and livestock can be predicted in various farming methods, such as using multiple classifier systems in ensemble learning or Bayesian models. The probabilistic graphical models encompassing Bayesian inference are used to investigate tasks with more incredible intricacy, like animal welfare measurement. Artificial intelligence systems utilising machine learning are quickly developing into ML-driven farms. Nowadays, machine learning focuses on particular problems, but when these technologies are joined into an interconnected system, farming practices will change to a system in which machine learning and data collection/analysis are essential.

4.2   MAJOR ACTIVITIES OF AGRICULTURE

4.2.1   Machine Learning in Agriculture

Machine learning is deeply involved in all stages of the growing and harvesting cycle. From preparing the soil to getting seeds to breed and determining the amount of water required for seed germination, the whole process begins with a seed planted in the ground. Finally, robots pick up the harvest and use computer vision to identify ripeness [4].

4.2.2   Species Management

4.2.2.1   Species Breeding

Overall, we have a favourable opinion of this application. Only harvest prediction and ambient conditions management are discussed as a late-stage application of the life cycle. Species selection is a lengthy process of searching for those particular genes that dictate many variables, including water and nutrient use, disease resistance, climate change adaptation and nutrient content. Over time, field research can allow machine learning and profound learning algorithms to discover a wide range of new information about crops and their performance under various climates and new characteristics discovered during the process. Since they have got the relevant data, they should use this data to create a probability model that would provide predictions on the genes that are most likely to contribute a valuable trait to a plant.

4.2.2.2 Species Recognition

With the conventional human approach to plant classification, comparing the colour and shape of leaves is used to arrive at plant classification. However, machine learning provides more accurate and faster results regarding leaf vein morphology because it carries more data about the leaf characteristics [5].

4.2.3 FIELD CONDITIONS MANAGEMENT

4.2.3.1 Soil Management

When it comes to farmers and agricultural specialists, the soil is a complex and diverse natural resource with ambiguous mechanisms at work. Researchers can better understand the impact of climate change on the local yield only by considering only the temperature. A computer model looks at the evaporation process, soil moisture and temperature to better understand the ecosystem dynamic behaviour and how it affects agriculture [6].

4.2.3.2 Water Management

Hydrological, climatological and agronomical balance are all significantly impacted by water management in agriculture. Due to ML-based applications, efficient irrigation system use is possible, leading to better weather forecasting and evapotranspiration prediction.

4.2.4 CROP MANAGEMENT

4.2.4.1 Yield Prediction

Precision agriculture is in consensus about yield prediction; concerning yield mapping and estimation, crop supply and demand tracking, and crop management, this issue is widely accepted. Comprehensive multidimensional analyses incorporating computer vision technologies provide a maximum yield for farmers and people in the population [7].

4.2.4.2 Crop Quality

Expanding on the benefits of accurately detecting and classifying crop quality characteristics, increasing product price and reducing waste all go hand in hand. Machines are better suited for dealing with seemingly insignificant data and interconnections because they can use them to provide helpful information about the crops, which may or may not be vital in terms of their overall quality [8].

4.2.4.3 Disease Detection

Because pesticides are generally sprayed evenly across the cropping area in both open-air and greenhouse conditions, the most commonly employed pest and disease control technique is uniform pesticide application. In order to be effective, the approach used here will require substantial amounts of pesticides, which ends up costing lots of money and incurring significant environmental harm. Agro-chemical input targeting the three types of variables, namely time, place and affected plants, is applied in precision agriculture management, also known as precision agriculture [9].

4.2.4.4 Weed Detection

In addition to illnesses, weeds are the main concern when it comes to crop yields. The greatest challenge in controlling weeds is that they are challenging to detect and identify from crops. Computer vision and machine learning algorithms can help weed detection and discrimination while minimising costs and zero effects on the environment. In the future, these technologies will most likely be used to develop weed-killing robots that require no herbicides [6].

4.2.5 Livestock Management

4.2.5.1 Livestock Production

In the same way that crop management helps farmers manage their fields, machine learning is applied to livestock production systems, such as cattle and egg production for helping in predicting and calculating farm parameters. For example, with systems that predict future weights, farmers can adjust their diets and conditions six months in advance, ensuring that their animals will not be overweight on the day they are slaughtered.

4.2.5.2 Animal Welfare

At present, livestock is seen as more than just edible resources. Farm animals are also recognised as having the potential to experience emotional distress, fatigue and even premature death on the farm. Animals' chewing patterns, when connected to diet changes, can let scientists know if a stressor was nearby and whether the animal is more or less likely to contract a disease. Animals that engage in chewing can reveal information such as whether or when the animal had recently encountered a stressor and whether it is more or less vulnerable to sickness, weight gain, and animal productivity [5].

Farmer's Little Helper is an app that serves as a bonus in the form of a last-minute dinner scenario. Imagine a farmer, exhausted after a long day, mustering the energy to decide the next steps in crop management. Which would sell more to a local farmer: to use for his business or participate in a regional agricultural event? Agricultural experts and companies are teaming up to build chatbots for farmers to communicate with them and provide them with information and data relevant to their needs.

While it is always intriguing to study the technologies that lay the groundwork for the future, the most critical aspect is how these technologies advance current technologies. Ascertaining what should be done through careful consideration and execution is a simple process, but developing and training machine learning models is a tricky task that requires both precise specification of input and results and constant iteration to produce novel predictions.

4.2.6 DRONE INVOLVEMENT IN AGRICULTURE

The UAV system is used to improve crop production and spray urea on the plant. Recent trends use plant monitoring, driven by the profits of many platforms in agriculture in particular. Spraying the area is necessary for plant growth management, and landing is based on the commands [10]. The UAV is used for calculating urea volume densities and the inspection of crops to minimise time and costs. It offers a rich and realistic feature that can satisfy the multiple requirements of the pesticide sprinkler. It also monitors crop growth and also provides multiple environmental features. The plant monitoring will provide reasonable estimates in both cost and flying lines. This implementation will increase the reliability of standard flying vehicles with new technology for production. The key objective is to improve quality and performance in high productivity, low power and high capacity. LiPo batteries can only be discharged at high levels [11].

In the previous method, the use of Arduino as a flight control board does not provide a specific rotation; it is not effective in rotating an engine, and we suggest a procedure to use ARM cortex m3 microcontroller to increase the function of the motor rotation. This work suggested a new quad-rotor model approach to spray urea in agriculture. It decreases farmers' labour and also improves field productivity in a short period. The UAV has a diameter of 1.8 m and can weigh up to 2 kg. It also consists of a sprayer with dust that can spray the urea at the transmitter's command. This work improves the UAV's weight elevation capacity, which can also spray sectorally. The UAV operates based on the relay driver and the transmitter commands [12].

4.3 BACKGROUND STUDY

There is extensive research in the machine learning field, but more deep knowledge has to be inferred when concerned with agriculture. Above all, working the drone with the former said is much more challenging in this era. Therefore, it is more important to have a suitable research methodology to go ahead further. The research made so far will be the stepping stone for all the authors who would like to bring flying colours into their proposals. The research made in all their idols known as DAD has to be made to support this chapter.

Rice (*Oryza sativa* L.) has been predicting the rice yields to control food inventory, which is in high demand globally. Mainly in China, rice makes up one-fifth of the total production. Climate variations impact the yield of crops. Eleven combinations of phenology, climate and geography data were tested for this study to predict the area-based crop yields using a primary regression-based method (MLR, multiple linear regression), and three ML methods: BP, SVM and random forest (RF). In conclusion, the MLR method was more precise. Only using critical parameters and geographic data that have been received yields improved results [13, 14].

A major role in agriculture is the planned use of animal manure, which regulates the farm-level law. They are fixed phosphorus (P) application forms. Once input and output are equal, an efficient manure application has been accomplished. The machine learning techniques are intended to predict production based on farm records and weather data. The dataset was previously used, and the regression model was used for model development. Since the data is limited, the prediction of P yield, and in addition to that, defining flexible P application norms before the first manure application are already feasible [15]. Thus, based on this assumption, the crop yield can be justified.

ML supports crop yield prediction to determine whether to grow a crop and which crop to cultivate [16]. A systematic literature review (SLR) for extracting and synthesising algorithms and features is presented to study the review. Fifty studies have been used to include the production analysis in the review. The most critical parameter is whether rainfall and soil type are applied to the ANN (artificial neural networks). LSTM and deep neural networks (DNN) are widely used in conjunction with CNNs (convolutional neural networks). Using text mining to classify the weather on Twitter automatically, with SVM, MNB and LR methods, SVM substantially outperforms various other machine learning algorithms for text classification, offering a classification accuracy of 93%. This means that SVM is ideal for text categorisation. We cluster the data to learn the restaurant's pattern in customers' opinions based on some measurement variables [17].

A thorough review of available techniques was conducted to develop grading and sorting techniques for dragon fruit, including CNN, ANN and SVM. These algorithms' work is based on the characteristics of dragon fruits, such as shape, size, weight, colour and disease [18]. By counting the total number of fruits available in the fruit bucket and using machine learning algorithms, raspberry functionality counts the number of fruits by maturity level [19].

The quadcopter, famously known as a drone, can freely monitor activities from remote locations. The article acts to incorporate these drones in various fields to monitor the action and predict some results [20]. The prediction will follow the scope of machine learning models in numerous application areas. The unmanned aerial vehicles and machine learning association have resulted in good results in many application areas, especially agriculture [21]. The proposed ground station architecture consists of drones and quadcopters, which have the primary function of monitoring and controlling the operations in all applications [22]. The data communication module, display module and digital map module are all created by them. The detailed design of the data communication module considers multi-threaded processing and the structural components of data. In addition to visualising data, the ground station provides several options for displaying data in the data display module, and a three-dimensional path planning method based on improved ant colony optimisation is proposed in the digital map module. The results of the experiment show that the ground station works well in real-time efficiency and durability.

M. K. Khan et al. have approached to design and develop a quadcopter for surveillance purposes, which incorporates many sub-modules for communication and management [10]. It has been purposely designed to automatically control the quadcopter by a flight controller APM2.7, which can be used for flight take-off and landing. The designed quadcopter has its specification with four brushless motors NTM 28–30 s 800 KV, and the Mobiousmini action camera with 1,080 MP is mounted to capture the live video and data are serially sent to the monitoring device for processing. The monitoring equipment is controlled by GPS Module N6N and Ublox 6 h GPS is placed on the quadcopter for proper navigation. It uses an Orange Rx T-Six 2.4 GHz transmitter for transmission of the navigational position feedback to the controller. Richard Steffen et al. have motivated the real-time capable vision system of a UAV for the trajectory and surface revamping of the aerial images sequences [11]. The challenge was to provide a real-time vision with a single camera to present the design and methods for the same. The initialisation process, map representation, estimation process, exploration strategies and loop closing detection were the various operations performed by the UAV. The critical point proposed was the Kalman filter used for the estimation process, followed by the landmark-based map representation with a new initialisation process and exploring strategy, finally contributing to a major impact on predicted camera trajectory and map accuracy. Landmark coordinates from a UAV without GPS was a complex challenge. The author added that future works can be applied with the sliding-window representation of the camera trajectory for better results in the approximation of motion in the Kalman filter rather than linear prediction models which were represented by orientations and corresponding velocities of the actual camera.

Ankith Shetty et al. proposed an approach to control a drone by just using the hand movements commonly known as hand gestures [13]. This paved the way for a human control interface to extract the ancient techniques of controlling using joysticks. This technique encourages more user-friendly human interaction with less knowledge of studying the instructions for controlling the different parameters of a drone. Unique algorithms are interfaced with different hand gesture input which was feasible only by employing image processing techniques using the webcam. This was implemented with the various modules incorporated, such as hand gesture capture and gesture monitor, feature extraction, and pattern matching for recognition of the gesture captured. Thus, this paper influenced an approach to control a quadcopter using gestures with the help of an Arduino and KK2.1.5 board.

An advanced unmanned aerial vehicle design has been tested for the safety and security of the industries. This vehicle is named the SWI 2020, which stands for safety wing for the industry in the year 2020. The system is to detect and locate intruders or unauthorised people entering into the security zone, which is interfaced with a unique board computer called Raspberry Pi. The quadcopter is equipped with a camera that detects and tracks unacceptable human movements with the help of Raspberry Pi, and live human activities are sent to the control station through Wi-Fi [23].

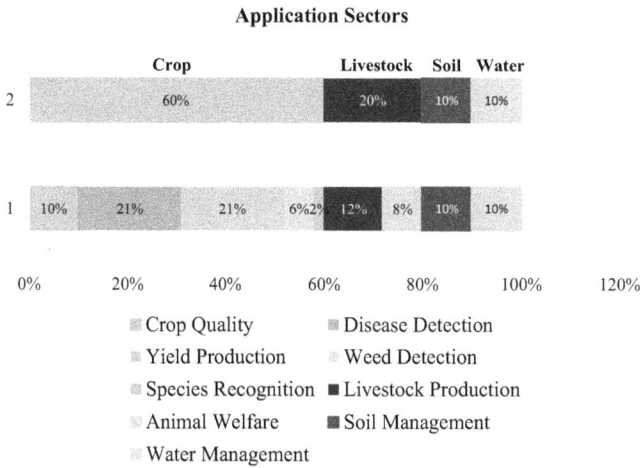

FIGURE 4.5 Articles distributed among application sectors.

4.4 EVALUATION

There was a variety of publications [13–21] in this study from various journals. Most of these publications focus on applications of machine learning in livestock production. Of those, the majority are focused on applications of machine learning in soil management. At the same time, the most significant number of them are related to crop quality and yield production. Figure 4.5 represents the articles that are distributed among different application sectors and classifications. According to the investigation of these articles, a total of eight machine learning techniques have been deployed. Notably, five machine learning techniques were used in crop management strategies, and four machine learning techniques were used in the livestock production area. Two machine learning techniques were used for water management.

Finally, four machine learning techniques were implemented in the soil management area. Figure 4.6 represents the rate of machine learning techniques.

Figure 4.7 represents the machine learning techniques for all publications based on the subcategory presented on the four main categories of crop, water, livestock and soil management. One of the most common machine learning models is an artificial neural network (ANN) and a support vector machine (SVM).

The subcategories' future technologies are detailed in Figure 4.8. These data show that multiple applications have been made using the ML techniques for crop and yield production (approximately 81 percent of them) and finding disease (21 percent). The distribution of the application of this agricultural pattern reveals that it incorporates extensive use of photos and data-intensive technologies. As a result, as an established scientific field, data analysis provides the foundation for developing a range of crop management applications that make use of machine learning (ML). Research findings revealed that the distribution of ML applications in livestock management (19 percent), water management (10 percent), and soil management (12 percent) could be partly explained by this (10 percent). Additionally, it was discovered

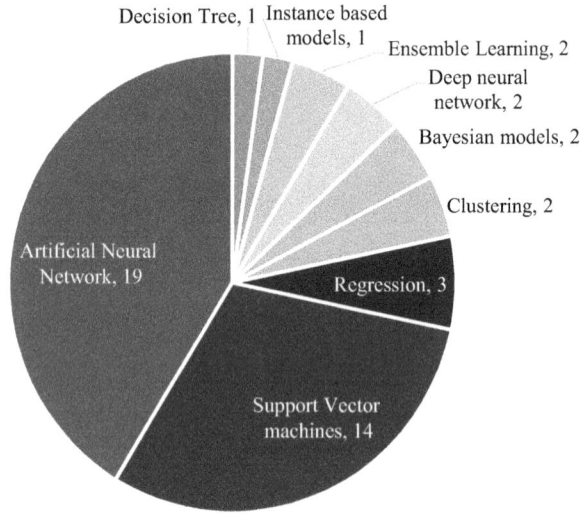

FIGURE 4.6   Rate of machine learning techniques.

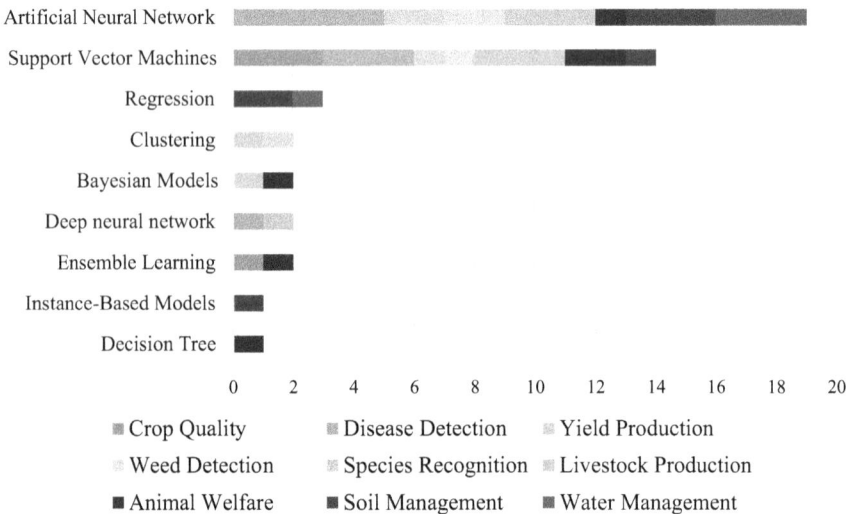

FIGURE 4.7   Machine learning techniques.

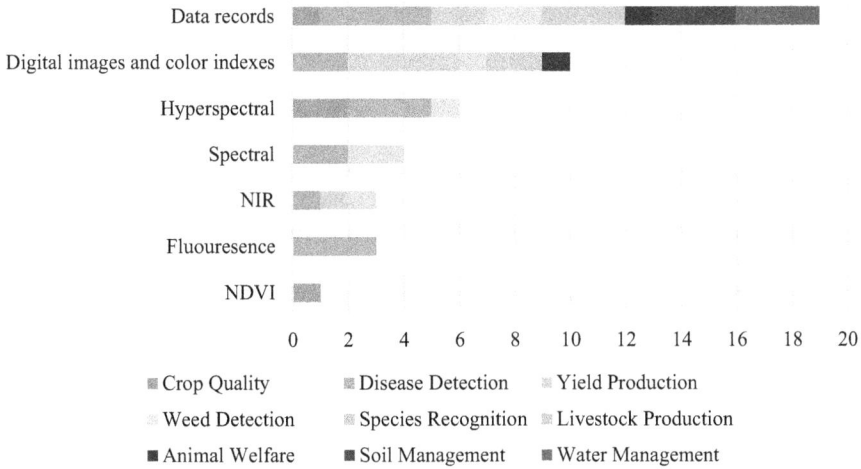

FIGURE 4.8   Data usage of resources.

that most of the studies utilised machine learning methods, including neural networks and support vector machines.

4.5   CASE STUDY: UREA SPRAYING IN AGRICULTURAL FIELDS USING UAV

Though there are many research areas in agriculture, a single application is focused on in a case study for the urea application in the agriculture field, subject to the chapter limitation. The research evaluation made 81 percent of machine learning concepts for crop quality and yield production more focused. SVM and ensemble models help concentrate on the crop quality, and the clustering, Bayesian, and ANN are focused on yield production. Thus, this case study focused on improving the crop quality by spraying urea in the lands wherever necessary based on the machine learning approach, which will be embedded in the Raspberry Pi connected with the urea sprayer microcontroller. Based on the learning, the drone will be moved to spray the urea for the proper yielding. Before controlling the drone, the machine learning algorithm commonly used, SVM, is embedded to perform its operation accordingly. As it is common usage in agriculture, more concentration is given to controlling the drone than to the machine learning algorithm in this case study.

Pesticides may have neurological effects, such as memory misfortune, lack of balance, reduced boost responses, diminished visual capacity, etc. In order to avoid the introduction of urea and welfare effects, the UAV is planned, which gives the ranchers and the field high productivity. The main goal of this mission is to resolve the awful consequences of the rancher's introduction to urea in the agricultural sector. The farmer should send instructions to the modified UAV so that the vehicle should swing according to the specified bearing. It will keep away from the evil effects and give farmers a good state of health. In general, several chemicals are introduced to the urea, which may affect the introduction of ranchers. Regarding the current system, the use of Arduino as a control board cannot offer a high degree of motor rotation specialisation, and temperature sensor cameras require high cost and lower performance. It can include radiometric and geometric calibrations and climate correction that is only possible from sensors in real-time. It also utilises remote sensing products with automotive rotation using fixed-wing UAV equipment and the commercial off-the-shelf technique (COTS) in that more than one lakh deaths are reported each year, in particular in developing world countries, due to human spraying pesticides and pesticides handling. Asthma, allergies and hypersensitivity are among the health effects of pesticides.

4.5.1 PROPOSED METHODOLOGY

Figure 4.9 shows the block diagram of the proposed drone. The ARM Cortex M3 microcontroller is used as a flight control board in this project as it is specialised in the rotation of the motor. This work uses the idea of a relay driver, which can serve as a switch. The controls are sent to the controller and then to the relay driver. When the relay is on, the dust sprays the urea, and the dust is closed, and the urea does not spray. This operates primarily on the thrust and air pressure in the propellers. The ARM cortex microcontroller is highly effective and powerful and can be used in real-time applications. It allows farmers to quickly turn the field by improving soil fertility and crop production. This implementation can require less expense and greater productivity than previous ideas and technologies. Quadcopter architecture [22] chips away with the norm of the high-weight transport of marvels.

The propellers force the air down with high weights, ensuring that creativity is limited and those movement reaction laws are usually related. These four propellers are attached to motors that move and cause the quadcopter to rise. The radio transmitter uses a radio flag to control the quadcopter remotely; the calls provided by the transmitter are received through a radio collector connected to the flight controller. The number of transmitters dictates how the pilot operates many flying machine activities. The quadcopter is an economical alternative to cost-prohibitive rotorcrafts. With fewer weighted parts, battery backup has been improved. Large payloads can be obtained in brushless BLDC-motors.

Using the proposed drone, Farmers are protected against poisons and heat strokes by sprayers on agricultural land of liquid pesticides, fertilisers, and herbicides. The proposed done has increased the profitability and yield of the product by showering the area evenly [24]. This device is also helpful in spraying pesticides from one location for a physically challenged farmer. With the farm drone, each species will operate continuously for 10–15 mins, each one-day surface area of each drone is 40–60 acres, the usage of pesticides is up by 40% or more, a lot of pesticides and energy are saved in comparison with conventional spraying techniques.

The initial prime application for this proposed model was to do surveillance in the industries. Later it was proposed to use it in the farms/lands. The drone developed will be the combination of both orthodox and outlook—the consideration of farming

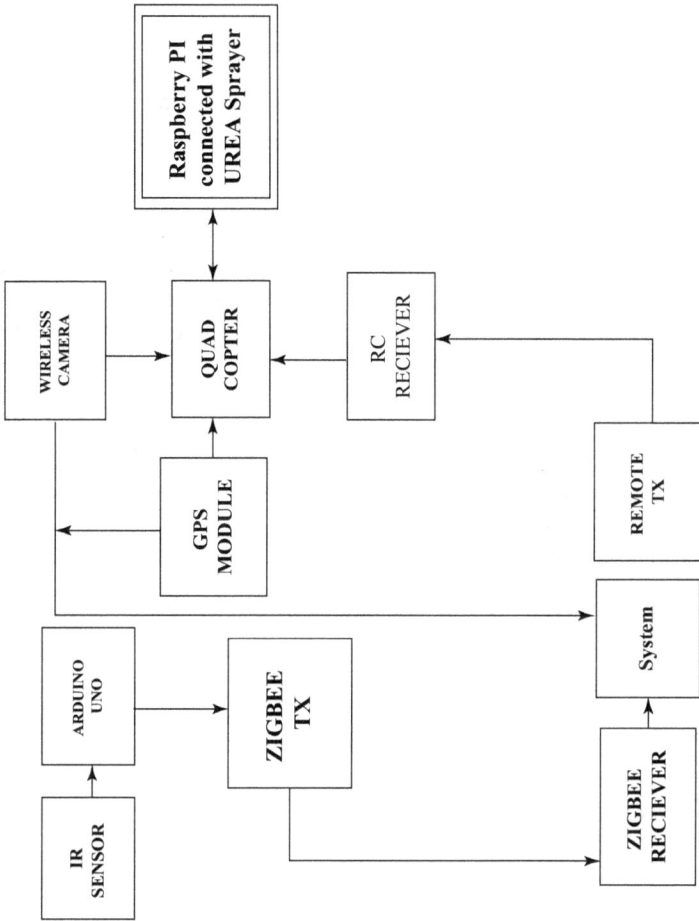

FIGURE 4.9 Architectural diagram of proposed drone.

in this proposal, which ultimately solves a standing farmer's problem over the years. The proposed drone can do urea spraying at multiple angles in a prodigious manner. Moreover, our motherland India is growing exponentially "digital", which creates the digital infrastructure, digital delivery services and digital literacy too which inter- and intraconnect our country with the rest of the world. The components used in the proposed model includes a drone damper—Electroprime 30X shock absorber (four pairs), landing gear—Tradico New Landing Gear (two pairs), landing gear—Tradico 65 mm Dia RC Airplane Plastic Hub Super Light Landing Gear Sponge Wheel (eight pairs), prop guard for drone production, drone's shell, accelerometer (two pairs), barometer (two pairs), gyroscope (two pairs), GPS (two pairs), drone motor—Brushless 1,100 kv (four units), prop mount with nut, washer and bolts (20 units), drone PCB with electronic speed controller, battery, UAV drone FPV&RPV, protector guard, spraying bottle, sprayer, rust-free stainless steel—Blade (16 units) and Audrino nanosensor (four units). Several applications are possible from the proposed UAV design, such as urea spraying, ecosystem management, wildlife research, precision agriculture and rangeland monitoring, security to chase down intruders, crack detection in dams and reactors and roof inspection in industries. A good architecture need not necessarily make a cognitive architecture. This statement boulevard a way to this research, which studies and implements the cognitive architecture for the intelligent drone. A cognitive architecture must be specific and derived from a general schema. It often incorporates relevant details, but it may include unnecessary elements as well. The use case, design and implementation choices will also determine whether or not it will have all the required elements. The use case design methodology concentrates on the concrete necessities of the cognitive architecture and on creating products based on user requirements [25].

Concerning this particular aspect, the goal here is concerned with developing an architecture that meets the demands of an application, even if it is inaccurate as a cognitive model. Accordingly, in this context, the architecture is more accurately viewed as conservative because it aims to preserve and maintain system-specific attributes and functions, which the system is capable of automatically discovering, anticipating, and carrying out, such as the capability to discern needs, anticipate actions and accomplish objectives. In this particular case, the design principles are not dictating the cognitive architecture—the requirements are doing that—but it helps to be aware of them to be aware of any potential capabilities and make an informed decision about whether or not to apply them. The concept of design by use case, in which routing the design through the meta-level schema is needed, is a concept with significant ramifications. A specific cognitive architecture is implied using a cognitive architecture schema at the meta-level abstracts. The particulars of the application that makes helpful are all facets of this approach.

4.6   CONCLUSION

A study dedicated to agricultural machine learning applications was previously reviewed in a more comprehensive review. Machine learning assists with all aspects of crop, livestock and water management. Smart farming, using drones with machine learning algorithms embedded within, is discussed in detail in this chapter. An intelligent evaluation has been made so that the researchers will have a glooming effect of applying machine learning in which areas of agriculture. The evaluation made supports to proceed further in-depth with the various machine learning technologies to take complete control of the farmers to support them in agriculture in all aspects. Further to that, a case study of integrating the drone, known as the unnamed vehicle, to perform its specific operation is done. This case study concentrates on how a drone can support the areas in agriculture, especially in the urea spraying application of the agricultural field. The study insists that a circuit system that includes the Raspberry Pi integrated with the urea spray controller is the interface between the control system and the drone. The SVM learning is embedded in the Raspberry Pi and the drone accordingly. Future studies may focus on the machine learning algorithm, which is more appropriate to work. Thus, an intelligent farming technology with the three idols DAD (drone agriculture deep learning) is proposed successfully.

REFERENCES

1. Sharma, Neha, Reecha Sharma, and Neeru Jindal. "Machine Learning and Deep Learning Applications-A Vision." *Global Transitions Proceedings* 2, no. 1 (2021): 24–28.
2. Guo, Yahui, Yongshuo Fu, Fanghua Hao, Xuan Zhang, Wenxiang Wu, Xiuliang Jin, Christopher Robin Bryant, and J. Senthilnath. "Integrated Phenology and Climate in Rice Yields Prediction Using Machine Learning Methods." *Ecological Indicators* 120 (2021): 106935.
3. Gaitán, Carlos F. "Machine Learning Applications for Agricultural Impacts under Extreme Events." In Jana Sillmann, Sebastian Sippel, and Simone Russo, editors. *Climate Extremes and Their Implications for Impact and Risk Assessment*, 119–138. Elsevier, 2020.
4. Dharmaraj, V., and C. Vijayanand. "Artificial Intelligence (AI) in Agriculture." *International Journal of Current Microbiology and Applied Sciences* 7, no. 12 (2018): 2122–2128.
5. Mollenhorst, Herman, Michel H. A. de Haan, Jouke Oenema, and Claudia Kamphuis. "Field and Crop Specific Manure Application on a Dairy Farm Based on Historical Data and Machine Learning." *Computers and Electronics in Agriculture* 175 (2020): 105599.
6. van Klompenburg, Thomas, Ayalew Kassahun, and Cagatay Catal. "Crop Yield Prediction Using Machine Learning: A Systematic Literature Review." *Computers and Electronics in Agriculture* 177 (2020): 105709.
7. Purwandari, Kartika, Join W. C. Sigalingging, Tjeng Wawan Cenggoro, and Bens Pardamean. "Multi-Class Weather Forecasting from Twitter Using Machine Learning Aprroaches." *Procedia Computer Science* 179 (2021): 47–54.
8. Patil, Pallavi U., Sudhir B. Lande, Vinay J. Nagalkar, Sonal B. Nikam, and G. C. Wakchaure. "Grading and Sorting Technique of Dragon Fruits Using Machine Learning Algorithms." *Journal of Agriculture and Food Research* 4 (2021): 100118.
9. Sambasivam, G., and Geoffrey Duncan Opiyo. "A Predictive Machine Learning Application in Agriculture: Cassava Disease Detection and Classification with Imbalanced Dataset Using Convolutional Neural Networks." *Egyptian Informatics Journal* 22, no. 1 (2021): 27–34.

10. Khan, M. K., A. Tauqir, H. Muazzam, and O. M. Butt. "Design of an Autonomous Surveillance Quad Copter." *Journal of Quality and Technology Management* 13, no. 1 (2016): 33–38.

11. Steffen, Richard, and Wolfgang Förstner. "On Visual Real Time Mapping for Unmanned Aerial Vehicles." In *21st Congress of the International Society for Photogrammetry and Remote Sensing (ISPRS)*, 57–62, 2008.

12. Shetty, Ankith, Archis Shinde, Jatin Patel, Nirav Panchal, and Martand Jha. "Gesture Controlled Quadcopter." *Imperial Journal of Interdisciplinary Research* 2, no. 5 (2016): 1289–1291.

13. Guo, Yahui, Yongshuo Fu, Fanghua Hao, Xuan Zhang, Wenxiang Wu, Xiuliang Jin, Christopher Robin Bryant, and J. Senthilnath. "Integrated Phenology and Climate in Rice Yields Prediction Using Machine Learning Methods." *Ecological Indicators* 120 (2021): 106935.

14. Sharma, Neha, Reecha Sharma, and Neeru Jindal. "Machine Learning and Deep Learning Applications-A Vision." *Global Transitions Proceedings* 2, no. 1 (2021): 24–28.

15. Mollenhorst, Herman, Michel H. A. de Haan, Jouke Oenema, and Claudia Kamphuis. "Field and Crop Specific Manure Application on a Dairy Farm Based on Historical Data and Machine Learning." *Computers and Electronics in Agriculture* 175 (2020): 105599.

16. van Klompenburg, Thomas, Ayalew Kassahun, and Cagatay Catal. "Crop Yield Prediction Using Machine Learning: A Systematic Literature Review." *Computers and Electronics in Agriculture* 177 (2020): 105709.

17. Purwandari, Kartika, Join W. C. Sigalingging, Tjeng Wawan Cenggoro, and Bens Pardamean. "Multi-Class Weather Forecasting from Twitter Using Machine Learning Aprroaches." *Procedia Computer Science* 179 (2021): 47–54.

18. Patil, Pallavi U., Sudhir B. Lande, Vinay J. Nagalkar, Sonal B. Nikam, and G. C. Wakchaure. "Grading and Sorting Technique of Dragon Fruits Using Machine Learning Algorithms." *Journal of Agriculture and Food Research* 4 (2021): 100118.

19. Sambasivam, G., and Geoffrey Duncan Opiyo. "A Predictive Machine Learning Application in Agriculture: Cassava Disease Detection and Classification with Imbalanced Dataset Using Convolutional Neural Networks." *Egyptian Informatics Journal* 22, no. 1 (2021): 27–34.

20. Khan, Asharul Islam, and Yaseen Al-Mulla. "Unmanned Aerial Vehicle in the Machine Learning Environment." *Procedia Computer Science* 160 (2019): 46–53.

21. Vij, Anneketh, Singh Vijendra, Abhishek Jain, Shivam Bajaj, Aashima Bassi, and Arushi Sharma. "IoT and Machine Learning Approaches for Automation of Farm Irrigation System." *Procedia Computer Science* 167 (2020): 1250–1257.

22. Liang, Xiao, Shirou Zhao, Guodong Chen, Guanglei Meng, and Yu Wang. "Design and Development of Ground Station for UAV/UGV Heterogeneous Collaborative System." *Ain Shams Engineering Journal* (2021). https://doi.org/10.1016/j.asej.2021.04.025.

23. Kumar, T. Ananth, S. Arunmozhi Selvi, R. S. Rajesh, and G. Glorindal. "Safety Wing for Industry (SWI 2020)–An Advanced Unmanned Aerial Vehicle Design for Safety and Security Facility Management in Industries." In G. Rajesh, X. Mercilin Raajini, and H. Dang, editors. *Industry 4.0 Interoperability, Analytics, Security, and Case Studies*, 181–198. CRC Press, 2021.

24. Raj, S. Gokul, N. Srinath, and T. Ananth Kumar. "Real-Time Trespasser Detection Using GPS Based UAV." In *2019 IEEE International Conference on Innovations in Communication, Computing and Instrumentation (ICCI)*, 50–54. IEEE, 2019.

25. John, A., T. Ananth Kumar, M. Adimoolam, and Angelin Blessy. "Energy Management and Monitoring Using IoT with CupCarbon Platform." In *Green Computing in Smart Cities: Simulation and Techniques*, 189–206. Springer, 2021.

5 Machine Learning and Deep Learning Paradigms and Case Studies

Sachit Mishra, Yash Joshi and R.S. Ponmagal

CONTENTS

5.1 IMAGING INVESTIGATION AND PROCESSING

The exploration of computer vision, image analytics and pattern acknowledgement has gained generous headway in the past few decades. Likewise, clinical imaging has pulled in expanding consideration lately because of its essential part in medical services applications.

Working along these lines to a natural eye, computer vision calculations discover examples and abnormalities in pictures to get a conclusion. Through a repetitive learning measure supported by neural networks, computer vision recognises, assesses and deciphers pictures.

5.1.1 CONVOLUTIONAL NEURAL NETWORKS

Picture-level diagnostics have been very effective at utilising CNN-based strategies. This is to a great extent because of the way that CNNs have accomplished

DOI: 10.1201/9781003132110-5

human-level execution in object-characterisation assignments, in which a CNN figures out how to order the article contained in a picture. CNN can be used in various fields of healthcare; for example, Rikiya Yamashita et al. [1] discussed how CNN can be used in radiology.

Advantages of convolutional neural networks include:

- *Accurate outcomes*: Computer vision frameworks offer exact analyses, limiting false positives. The innovation can possibly demolish the prerequisite for repetitive surgeries and costly treatments. Computer vision calculations prepared utilising a colossal measure of training information can recognise the smallest presence of a condition that may commonly be ignored by human specialists due to their tactile impediments. The utilisation of computer vision in medical services determination can give altogether undeniable degrees of exactness which may in coming time go up to 100%. In any event, when human clinicians were furnished with foundation data on patients, like age, sex and the body site of the presume include, the CNN beat the dermatologists by almost 7%.
- *Clinical imaging*: In the past few years, computer vision upheld clinical imaging application has been dependable assistance for doctors. It doesn't just make and break down pictures, yet additionally turns into a partner and assists specialists with their understanding. The application is utilised to peruse and change over 2D output pictures into intelligent 3D models that empower clinical experts to acquire a definite comprehension of a patient's ailment.
- *Early identification of ailment*: Numerous lethal infections, for example, malignancy, should be analysed at a beginning phase to expand the odds of endurance of the patient. Computer vision has been widely used for the early identification of these sicknesses. Computer vision empowers the location of early manifestations with high conviction inferable from its finely tuned design acknowledgement capacity. This can be helpful for convenient treatment and saving innumerable lives as long as possible.
- *Increased medical process*: The utilisation of computer vision in medical care can impressively reduce the time specialists take in examining reports and pictures. It liberates and offers them more opportunity to go through with patients and give customised and valuable guidance. By upgrading the nature of doctor–patient associations, it can likewise help clinical experts to offer conferences to an ever-increasing number of patients. The utilisation of computer vision in medical care upholds health workers to convey productive and precise medical services administrations through its life-saving applications.
- *Nuclear medication*: As a part of clinical medication, atomic medication manages the utilisation of radionuclide drugs in finding. Now and again computer vision procedures of distant radiation treatment additionally allude to atomic medication. In diagnostics, it predominantly uses single-photon emanation processed tomography and positron discharge tomography.

5.1.2 Use Cases

- *Lung cancer detection*:
  Jeyaprakash Vasanth Wason et al. [2] proposed a system for early identification of lung cancer using computer-aided diagnosis and computed tomography (CT) scan.

  - *The process*:
    The initial step is pre-handling of the picture to find particles utilising force measure. The handled picture is portioned utilising a standard division method. Subsequently, malignant growth knobs are set apart in the picture. Notwithstanding highlights like region, edge and unconventionality, different highlights like centroid, measurement and pixel mean force have been removed during feature extraction.

    Extracted features are utilised as training instances and the relating prepared model is created for the grouping followed by model assessment for identification and order with improved exactness, explicitness and affectability.

  - *Outcome*:
    1. Better exactness of malignancy knob identification.
    2. Groups the identified cellular breakdown in the lungs as malignant or benign.
    3. Eliminates the clamours that make incorrect identification of disease.

- *Brain tumour detection*:
  Sahithi Ankireddy et al. [3] proposed a process to detect brain tumours using a Mask R convolutional neural network to increase the accuracy of diagnosis.

  - *The process*:
    In order to acquire pre-trained instances from Mask R CNN, transfer learning was used. The Mask R CNN setup was broadened, and boundaries were changed to coordinate with the tumour identification issue. Then, the Mask R CNN dataset class was stretched out to execute certain strategies, for example, stacking the CT scan dataset, cover and so on. After the essential advances were finished, the model was set up to be prepared. The model catalogue, loads and arrangement were assembled. The module was trained over 20 epochs.

  - *Outcome*:
    The forecast division coordinated at 90% with the ground truth. This recommends that the model had the option to perform at an undeniable level.

5.2 DRUG INVENTION AND PRECISION MEDICATION

Accuracy of medication and medication revelation are additionally on the plan for deep learning engineers. The two errands require treating really gigantic volumes of genomic, clinical and populace-level information to recognise the heretofore obscure relationship between qualities, drugs and actual conditions.

Deep learning is a perfect methodology for analysts and drug partners hoping to feature new instances in these moderately neglected informational indexes—particularly in light of the fact that numerous precision medication scientists don't yet know precisely the thing they ought to be searching for.

Medication revelation is one of the spaces that can acquire an advantage from the achievement of deep learning. Medication disclosure is a tedious and costly assignment and deep learning can be utilised to make this cycle quicker and less expensive.

Drug discovery is a long and expensive process that generally includes the following steps:

1. Discovery
2. Pre-clinical trial
3. Clinical trial
4. Regulatory approval
5. Mass production

The expected effect of deep learning in drug revelation includes how artificial intelligence can be utilised to eliminate the time spent on drug disclosure, utilising its capacity to dissect enormous volumes of clinical information to recognise examples and associations with more prominent viability than people. Since a significant piece of the underlying medication disclosure tests depends on experimentation, deep learning calculations can be utilised to reproduce and precisely study the impacts of different synthetic substances on the objective microorganisms, through virtual high-throughput screening.

Lauv Patel et al. [4] in their paper discussed the various machine learning methods that can be used in drug invention or discovery, including precision medication.

The desire of precision medication is to plan and advance the pathway for finding remedial mediation, and guess by utilising enormous multidimensional organic datasets that catch singular inconstancy in qualities, capacity and climate. This offers healthcare workers the chance to all the more cautiously tailor early mediations.

Exploiting elite system capacities, artificial intelligence (AI) calculations would now be able to make sensible progress in foreseeing hazards in specific malignancies and cardiovascular infection from accessible multidimensional clinical and natural information.

Deep learning is now also making some progress in the field of neurodevelopmental disorders like epilepsy and autism. Mohammed Uddin et al. [5] has explained this in detail in their paper.

AI calculations can make an effect in complex uncertain issues in neurodevelopmental disorders such as:

- *Recognising causal genes*: AI techniques are urgent for distinguishing causal qualities and loci. Bioinformatics forecast is still not ready to precisely group the more normal disorders' transformations according to pathogenicity. In any event, recognising causal qualities from those "varieties of uncertain significance" (VUS) stays a significant uncertain issue that fits an AI arrangement.
- *Genetic and phenotypic heterogeneity*: Over the past few years, digitisation of clinical wellbeing records added a lot of information identified with medical care. The use of AI calculations may be essentially profitable to those digitisation endeavours that can help set up genotype aggregate connections for hereditary illnesses and have the ability to finish up various phenotypic relationships and affiliations.
- *Gene–gene interactions and polygenic risk score*: Gene–gene connection is a significant supporter of the phenotypic change of NDDs; however, there is right now no tenable AI calculation ready to adapt to information on this scale. There exist significant intricacies concerning profound phenotypic and huge-scope omics information. Solo AI approaches might be applied to see beforehand obscure sub-structures inside NDD cases dependent on natural elements, measurements balance, and so on.

5.2.1   USE CASES

- *Accelerating the process of drug discovery*:
  Zhihong Liu et al. [6] in their paper explained how we can use deep learning for a screening web service to reduce the time taken in the process of drug discovery.

  Deep learning contributes altogether to investigations in organic sciences and medication disclosure. Past examinations proposed that deep learning methods have shown better execution than other machine learning calculations in virtual screening, which is a basic advance to speed up the medication disclosure.

  - *The process*:
    The structure of a deep-learning-oriented virtual screening service consists of the following:
    1. Data index preparation: select an objective of interest, or transfer a private data index for deep neural network (DNN) preparation.
    2. Attributes: select attributes for atomic vectorisation.
    3. Boundaries: select model boundaries for preparing characterisation or relapse models.
    4. Implicit screening: implicit screening against a synthetic library or a new library.

- *Outcome*:
  The normal and middle of AUC were 0.89 and 0.86, individually, which demonstrates a decent screening execution of those developed deep learning applications.

5.3 PREDICTIVE ANALYSIS AND CLINICAL DECISION ASSISTANCE

The world has high expectations for the part of deep learning in predictive analysis and clinical decision assistance for a wide assortment of conditions.

Deep learning may before long be a helpful indicative partner in the inpatient setting, where it can make suppliers aware of changes in high-hazard conditions like respiratory breakdown and sepsis. AI strategies are best-in-class in prescient demonstration in fields like computer vision and self-ruling routes. Progressively, these devices are utilised for clinical prescient demonstrating and clinical support help, where clinical qualities are utilised to anticipate a clinical status like a result or a hazard.

Notwithstanding, a typical analysis of these advanced methods is that while they may build model execution they don't give the likelihood to clarify the subsequent forecasts. Conversely, customary methods permit clarifications by different methods and this methodology has been the foundation of logical clinical prescient demonstrating to date.

Luckily, interpretability strategies customised to current machine learning calculations have arisen of late, in this way conceivably permitting elite and reasonable models. For one, in the most recent couple of years, a few methods have been created to open the most infamous black box, to be specific artificial neural networks and give logical models.

Stefania Montani et al. [7] in their work discussed how clinical decision assistance frameworks desire to improve judgement-making, with the end goal to enhance the nature of care given by medical care associations.

5.3.1 USE CASES

- *Non-invasive forecast of diabetes*:
  Sebastian Spänig et al. [8] has discussed in length how deep learning can be used for the non-invasive forecast of diabetes.

  A huge number of individuals are treated in trauma centres in medical clinics consistently. In any case, a critical number of the patients are non-crisis cases, constraining the clinics to allot the clinical workforce where it isn't really required, making a problematic utilisation of staff and treatment of genuine patient crises.

  In addition, there is a developing inadequacy of doctors in rustic regions, prompting underserved patients, specifically, because of the segment change and a developing number of old individuals.

  One answer to tackle these issues may be the utilisation of artificial intelligence in medical services as a driver for frameworks medication.

- *The process*: The end goal of the study is:
  1. The improvement of an AI ready to cooperate with a patient (virtual specialist).
  2. To exhibit its helpfulness on the mechanised forecast of a model infection, to be specific T2DM, on a huge patient associate.
  3. The plan and investigation of a poll on the acknowledgement of AI in medication by youthful grown-ups.

- *Outcome*:
  The DNN prepared without HbA1c beats the SVM as far as AUC. DNN and SVM show comparative expectation execution when used with HbA1c.

- *Spine oncology study*:
  Elie Massaad et al. [9] discussed how predictive analysis can be used in spine oncology study. The capability of huge information investigation to improve the nature of care for patients with spine tumours is critical. Right now, the utilisation of enormous information examination for oncology and spine medical procedure is at an incipient stage. Accordingly, endeavours are in progress to propel information-driven oncologic consideration, improve patient results and guide clinical dynamics.

  This is both important and basic in the act of spine oncology as clinical dynamic is frequently made in separation, taking a look at select factors considered applicable by the doctor. With quickly advancing therapeutics in medical procedures, radiation, interventional radiology and oncology, there is a need to more readily create dynamic calculations using the immense information accessible for every patient.

  - *The process*:
    Artificial intelligence (AI) is a part of software engineering that intends to create instruments that can take the abilities of human intelligence and even outflank human undertakings while investigating big data. Artificial intelligence designing alludes to the overall capacity to plan programming/machines that freely imitate the scholarly cycles of human cognisance in settling on an activity because of its apparent climate to accomplish a foreordained objective. In spine medical procedures, AI is as of now being utilised in radiologic findings, careful arranging and result forecast.

  - *Outcome*:
    The field of AI is continually growing, driven by progress in innovation and software engineering. Data keeps on being the most essential segment for learning AI frameworks and applying such frameworks to the field of spine oncology is in its earliest stages.

5.4   NATURAL LANGUAGE PROCESSING

Deep learning and neural organisations as of now support a large number of the natural language processing devices that have gotten well known in the medical services industry for directing documentation and making an interpretation of discourse-to-message.

The selection of natural language processing in medical care is rising as a result of its perceived potential to look, examine and decipher mammoth measures of patient datasets. Utilising progressed clinical calculations, AI in medical care and NLP innovation administrations can possibly outfit important experiences and ideas from information that was recently viewed as covered in text structure.

NLP in medical services media can precisely offer a voice to the unstructured information of the medical care universe, giving fantastic knowledge into getting quality, improved strategies and better outcomes for patients.

Physicians spend a lot of time inputting the how and the why of what's happening to their patients into chart notes. These notes aren't effectively extractable in manners the information can be investigated by a figure. When the medical professional sits down with you, and make notes of your visit in a case note, those narratives go into the electronic health record systems and get stored as free text.

Medical care natural language processing utilises particular motors fit for scouring enormous arrangements of unstructured wellbeing information to find recently missed or inappropriately coded patient conditions. Natural language processing clinical records utilising machine-learned calculations can reveal infection that might not have been recently coded, a vital element for making HCC illness disclosures.

In the beginning, with regards to medical services, the innovation has two use cases:

- Understanding human discourse and separating its importance.
- Opening unstructured information in datasets and archives by delineating fundamental ideas and values and permitting doctors to utilise this data for dynamic and investigation.

All extra use instances of AI and NLP in medical services will grow out of these two essential elements of the innovation.

Improvement in clinical documentation: AI in medical services has contacted clinical documentation, opening up doctors from the manual and complex design of EHRs, permitting them to focus more on care conveyance.

Speech recognition: NLP has developed its utilisation case in discourse acknowledgement throughout the years by permitting clinicians to decipher notes for helpful EHR information passage.

Computer-assisted coding: NLP-driven CAC vows to improve coder exactness. PC-aided coding separates data about strategies and treatments to catch each code and augment claims.

Data mining research: the reconciliation of information mining in medical care frameworks permits associations to diminish the degrees of subjectivity in dynamics and give helpful clinical skills.

Sumithra Velupillai et al. [10] in their work has discussed how the significance of medical NLP has been on the rise for the past few years and how it has led to some path-breaking advances.

5.4.1 Use Cases

• *Medical text analysis of chronic diseases*:
  Seyedmostafa Sheikhalishahi et al. [11] in their paper have highlighted how NLP can be used to investigate and draw outcomes from medical text.

  • *The process*:
    Favoured reporting articles system review and meta-analyses rules were followed and attention was directed to five data indexes utilising "medical notes", "natural language processing" and "persistent illness" and their varieties as catchphrases to augment inclusion of the articles.

  • *Outcome*:
    Endeavours are yet needed to improve:
    1. Movement of clinical NLP strategies from extraction toward understanding.
    2. Acknowledgement of relations among substances as opposed to elements in seclusion.
    3. Fleeting extraction to comprehend past, current and future clinical occasions.
    4. Misuse of elective wellsprings of clinical information.

5.5 AI-ASSISTED RADIOLOGY AND PATHOLOGY

These days, electronically set aside clinical imaging data is extensive and DL computations can be used to deal with such a dataset, to recognise and discover models and peculiarities. Machines and estimations can unravel the imaging data comparable as a particularly arranged radiologist could—perceiving questionable spots on the skin, wounds, tumours and brain channels. The usage of AI/ML instruments/stages for aiding radiologists is, as such, readied to develop drastically.

They are depended upon to overhaul the idea of motorisation and savvy dynamics in fundamental/tertiary patient thought and public clinical consideration structures. This could be the best impact of AI devices as it can change the individual fulfilment for billions of people all through the planet.

Artificial intelligence (AI) computations, particularly significant learning, have shown great headway in picture affirmation tasks. Procedures going from convolutional neural associations to varying autoencoders have found bundle applications in the clinical picture examination field, driving it forward at a quick speed. Really, in radiology practice, arranged specialists apparently studied clinical pictures for the area, depiction and seeing of diseases. AI procedures overwhelm at normally seeing complex models in imaging data and giving quantitative, instead of emotional, examinations of radiographic characteristics.

5.5.1 Use Cases

- *Use of AI in pathology*:
  An astounding test is "Microsoft's Project InnerEye" which uses ML methodologies to partition and recognise tumours using 3D radiological pictures. It can help in precise operation masterminding, course and beneficial tumour-moulding for radiotherapy organising.

  ML instruments are also adding gigantic worth by expanding the expert's feature with information, for instance, danger limitation during mechanical frameworks and other picture-guided interventions. The utilisation of AI/ML instruments/stages for aiding radiologists is, accordingly, arranged to develop significantly.

  As referred to by Shihab Sarwar [12], overall, respondents passed on usually elevating points of view towards AI, with practically 75% itemising income or energy in AI as a definite device to work with upgrades in work measure capability and quality affirmation in pathology.

  Degrees of progress in PC vision and artificial intelligence (AI) pass on the likelihood of making basic responsibilities to clinical consideration, particularly in suggestive strengths like radiology and pathology. The impact of these developments on specialist accomplices is the subject of enormous theory.

  There is, at any rate, inadequacy of information as for the speculations, excitement and stresses of disease and illness development.

  Results from an outline of 487 pathologist-respondents practising in 54 countries were coordinated to examine perspectives on AI execution in clinical practice.

  Despite limitations, fusing issues with estimating response tendency and checking the character of respondents to this obscure and intentional outline, a couple of interesting revelations were uncovered.

- *Thoracic imaging*:
  Cellular breakdown in the lungs is perhaps the most well-known and dangerous sign of tumours. Screening of cellular breakdown in the lungs can help recognise aspiratory knobs, with early identification being lifesaving in numerous patients. Artificial intelligence (AI) can help in naturally distinguishing these knobs and ordering them as kind or harmful.

- *Artificial intelligence in radiology*:
  There are two strategies for utilising AI in medication:
  1. *AI*:
     Conventional artificial intelligence (AI) techniques depend to a great extent on predefined designed element calculations with express boundaries dependent on master information. Such highlights are intended to evaluate explicit radiographic attributes, for example, the 3D state of a tumour or the intratumoral surface and dissemination of pixel powers (histogram).

A resulting choice advance guarantees that solitary the most important highlights are utilised. Factual AI models are then fitted to this information to distinguish potential imaging-based biomarkers.

Instances of these models incorporate help vector machines and arbitrary woodlands.

2. *Deep learning*:

Ongoing advances in AI research have brought about new, non-deterministic, deep learning calculations that don't need unequivocal component definition, addressing a generally extraordinary worldview in AI.

The basic strategies for deep learning have existed for quite a long time. Be that as it may, just lately have adequate information and computational force become accessible.

Without unequivocal component predefinition or choice, these calculations adapt straightforwardly by exploring the information space, giving them unrivalled critical thinking capacities.

- *Brain imaging*:
Brain tumours are depicted by surprising advancement of tissue and can be benign, hazardous, fundamental or metastatic; AI could be used to make definite figures [13].

5.6 ELECTRONIC HEALTH RECORDS

Even more actually deep learning has been applied to deal with amassed EHRs, including both coordinated (for instance, medications, research office tests) and unstructured (for instance, free-text clinical notes) data. The best piece of this composing arranged the EHRs of a clinical benefits system with a deep plan for a specific, ordinarily supervised, perceptive clinical endeavour.

In particular, a regular technique is to show that deep learning gets the best results over standard AI models concerning explicit estimations, similar to area under the receiver operating characteristic curve, exactness and F-score.

In the present circumstance, while most papers present beginning-to-end supervised associations, a couple of works in like manner propose unsupervised models to induce dormant patient depictions, which are then surveyed using shallow classifiers (for instance, sporadic forests, vital backslide).

RNNs with long short-term memory (LSTM) concealed units, pooling and word embeddings were used in DeepCare [14], a beginning-to-end deep incredible association that interprets momentum infection states and predicts future clinical outcomes.

The makers furthermore proposed to coordinate the LSTM unit with a decay effect to manage inconsistent arranged events (which are normal in longitudinal EHRs). Also, they joined clinical interventions in the model to logically shape the assumptions.

DeepCare was surveyed for sickness development illustrating, intercession proposition and future risk conjecture on diabetes and passionate prosperity patient associates.

Deep learning was also applied to show unending time signals, for instance, lab results, near the customised unmistakable confirmation of unequivocal totals.

For example, Lipton et al. [15] used RNNs with LSTM to see plans in a multivariate time course of action of clinical assessments.

Specifically, they arranged a model to orchestrate 128 discoveries from 13 different sources to identify the factors from patients in pediatric concentrated unit care.

5.7 ROBOT-ASSISTED SURGERY

Concerning potential, robot-helped surgery is at the highest point of the AI-engaged class. Artificial intelligence–enabled progressed mechanics can improve and deal with the exactness of the cautious instrument by planning consistent working estimations, data from genuine cautious experiences, and information from pre-activity clinical records. Surely, Accenture reports that these advances made possible by AI-engaged mechanical innovation fuse a length of stay diminished by 21%.

Inspecting various plans, I find Mazor Robotics for the most part promising. It is using AI to restrict the meddling and intensify the customisation of cautious strategy on domains with complex life frameworks—like the spine. The AI structure helps the expert arrangement where supplements will be put using CT analyses before the patient is accessible, and Mazor's robot arm for spinal surgery coordinates the advancement of the cautious instruments, ensuring a genuine degree of precision.

There have certainly been occurrences of over-promoted developments, but AI is by no means whatsoever among them.

Undoubtedly, even as we stay at the early edge of the development, with its potential just hardly fathomed, the clinical care industry is experiencing an upsurge of effectiveness and pay due to AI.

Most critical clinical consideration players are currently placing assets into AI, seeing huge pieces of this advancement later for the business. Where it takes us from here will be invigorating to see; in any case, an overall instructed, considered appraisal with the right data will have the clearest chance concerning predicting its direction.

As referred to by Jyotsna Dwivedi [16], computerised surgery has been around for over 20 years, and has been a reformist development in improving medical procedures. The usage of cutting-edge mechanics in activities has become essential in the earlier decade.

With the wide affirmation in mechanised surgery, the drive to give more humble, more profitable and more moderate equipment is driving experts to show up at fantastic heights. Mechanised surgery has been adequately completed in a couple of crisis facilities all through the planet and has gotten, generally speaking, affirmation.

The articulation "robot" was conceived by Karel Capek, who was a Czech essayist. The source comes from the root "robota", which means compelled work like the machines that do repeated, unassuming work.

Unimportantly, meddlesome surgery moreover has its obstructions. A segment of the more prominent cutoff points incorporates the particular and mechanical nature of the equipment. Experts found it somewhat difficult to control the instruments while watching a 2D picture.

The medical robots of today started from the 1985 robot, Programmable Universal Manipulation Arm (PUMA) 560 used by Kwoh.

In the last decade alone, various tools are availabe for finding out the results and also maintaining the similarity index according to that.

While cost has been an issue concerning the arrangement and improvement of the robots, the money-related feasibility of this endeavour has controlled the blazes of various mechanical experts all through the planet.

A critical number of the medical robots used in the forefront of surgery find their beginnings in the gatekeeper and business market. With movements in broadcast interchanges, the ascent of subfields in remote medicine, such as telesurgery, has taken the front line.

Computerised surgery may have a long approach, yet it has successfully exhibited its worth according to various clinical masters as well as patients all around the planet.

Despite the way that the learning curve for these structures is to some degree steep, there is no doubt that this is the cautious development of what might be on the horizon.

In the new progressed age, with the astounding advancement of development, the next decade pledges to bring significantly more important, more modest, adaptable and accurate medical structures.

A couple of mechanical structures are at present certified by the FDA for express medical procedures. As referred to previously, ROBODOC is used to precisely focus out the femur in hip replacement surgery.

PC Motion Inc. of Goleta, CA, has two systems accessible. One, called AESOP, is a voice-controlled endoscope with seven degrees of chance.

This structure can be used in any laparoscopic strategy to overhaul the expert's ability to control a consistent picture.

The Zeus structure and the Da Vinci system have been used by a combination of orders for laparoscopic operations, including cholecystectomies, mitral valve fixes, radical prostatectomies, reversal of tubal ligations, despite various gastrointestinal operations, nephrectomies and kidney transplants.

The number and kinds of operations being performed with robots are growing rapidly as more establishments secure these structures.

Perhaps the most striking use of these structures, regardless, is in totally endoscopic coronary vein joining, a framework that was some time ago outside the limitations of laparoscopic advancement.

5.8 PERSONALISED TREATMENT AND BEHAVIOURAL MODIFICATION

Between 2012 and 2017, the uptake rate of electronic health records in healthcare rose from 40% to 67%.

This typically infers more permission to solitary patient health data.

By organising this individual clinical data of individual patients with ML applications and computations, healthcare providers (HCPs) can recognise and overview health.

Considering supervised learning, clinical specialists can predict the perils and threats to a patient's health as demonstrated by the signs and inherited information in their clinical history.

As referred to by Sunil Mathur [17], personalised medicine (PM) is connected to making a therapy as individualised as the affliction. Data on PM works with earlier affliction acknowledgement through redesigned usage of existing biomarkers and area of early genomic and epigenomic events in ailment progression, particularly carcinogenesis.

The philosophy relies upon perceiving innate, epigenomic and clinical information that allows the jump advances in our cognisance of how a person's excellent genomic portfolio makes them vulnerable to explicit disorders.

The PM approach is a completed expansion of standard technique (one-size-fits-all) to extend our ability to predict which clinical medications will be ensured and effective for solitary patients, and which ones will not be, based on the patient's unique genetic profile.

Execution of PM can reduce expenditure and time utilisation, and in addition, increase individual fulfilment and lifespan of patients.

Extending healthcare costs have put additional pressure on government upheld healthcare systems from one side of the planet to the other, especially for end-of-life care.

PM is seen as headway in the healthcare system; it is preventive, synchronised and illustrated.

PM can offer improved solution assurance and zero in on treatment, diminish hostile effects, increase patient consistency, move the target of drug from reaction to aversion, and improve cost sufficiency.

REFERENCES

1. Yamashita, R., Nishio, M., Do, R., & Togashi, K. (2018, August). Convolutional neural networks: An overview and application in radiology. Retrieved May 01, 2021, from https://www.ncbi.nlm.nih.gov/pmc/articles/PMC6108980/
2. Wason, J., & Nagarajan, A. (2019, September 12). Image processing techniques for analyzing CT scan images towards the early detection of lung cancer. Retrieved May 01, 2021, from https://www.ncbi.nlm.nih.gov/pmc/articles/PMC6822523/
3. Ankireddy, S. (2020). Assistive Diagnostic Tool for Brain Tumor Detection using Computer Vision. arXiv preprint arXiv:2011.08185.
4. Patel, L., Shukla, T., Huang, X., Ussery, D. W., & Wang, S. (n.d.). Machine learning methods in drug discovery. Retrieved May 01, 2021, from https://pubmed.ncbi.nlm.nih.gov/33198233/
5. Uddin, M., Wang, Y., & Woodbury-Smith, M. (2019, November 21). Artificial intelligence for precision medicine in neurodevelopmental disorders. Retrieved May 01, 2021, from https://www.nature.com/articles/s41746-019-0191-0
6. Liu, Z., Du, J., Fang, J., Yin, Y., Xu, G., & Xie, L. (2019, October 11). DeepScreening: A deep learning-based screening web server for accelerating drug discovery. Retrieved May 01, 2021, from https://academic.oup.com/database/article/doi/10.1093/database/baz104/5585580?login=true

7. Montani, S., & Striani, M. (2019, August). Artificial intelligence in clinical decision support: A focused literature survey. Retrieved May 01, 2021, from https://www.ncbi .nlm.nih.gov/pmc/articles/PMC6697510/

8. Spänig, S., Emberger-Klein, A., Sowa, J.-P., Canbay, A., Menrad, K., & Heider, D. (2019). The virtual doctor: An interactive artificial intelligence based on deep learning for non-invasive prediction of diabetes. Artif Intell Med. 100, 101706. 10.1016/j. artmed.2019.101706. Epub 2019 Aug 21. PMID: 31607340.

9. Massaad, E., Fatima, N., Hadzipasic, M., Alvarez-Breckenridge, C., Shankar, G., & Shin, J. (2019, December). Predictive analytics in spine oncology research: First steps, limitations, and future directions. Retrieved May 01, 2021, from https://www.ncbi.nlm .nih.gov/pmc/articles/PMC6944986/

10. Velupillai, S., Suominen, H., Liakata, M., Roberts, A., Shah, A., Morley, K., ... & Dutta, R. (2018, October 24). Using clinical natural language processing for health outcomes research: Overview and actionable suggestions for future advances. Retrieved May 01, 2021, from https://www.sciencedirect.com/science/article/pii/S1532046418302016#:~ :text=Within%20EHR%20systems%2C%20NLP%2   0may,information%20in%20a %20patient's%20record.&text=Tools%20such%20as%20Turf%20(EHR,soluti ons%20for% 20clinical%20research%20problems.

11. Sheikhalishahi, S., Miotto, R., Dudley, J., Lavelli, A., Rinaldi, F., Osmani, V., ... & Osmani, C. (n.d.). Natural language processing of clinical notes on chronic diseases: Systematic review. Retrieved May 01, 2021, from https://medinform.jmir.org/2019/2/ e12239/

12. Hosny, A., Parmar, C., Quackenbush, J., Schwartz, L., & Aerts, H. (2018, August). Artificial intelligence in radiology. Retrieved May 01, 2021, from https://www.ncbi.nlm .nih.gov/pmc/articles/PMC6268174/

13. Orringer, D., Pandian, B., Niknafs, Y., Hollon, T., Boyle, J., Lewis, S., ... & Camelo-Piragua, S. (2017). Rapid intraoperative histology of unprocessed surgical specimens via fibre-laser-based stimulated Raman scattering microscopy. Retrieved May 01, 2021, from https://www.ncbi.nlm.nih.gov/pmc/articles/PMC5612414/

14. Miotto, R., Wang, F., Wang, S., Jiang, X., & Dudley, J. (2018, November 27). Deep learning for healthcare: Review, opportunities and challenges. Retrieved May 01, 2021, from https://www.ncbi.nlm.nih.gov/pmc/articles/PMC6455466/#bbx044-B58

15. Lipton, Z., Kale, D., Elkan, C., & Wetzel, R. (2015). Learning to diagnose with LSTM recurrent neural networks.

16. Jyotsna, D., & Mahgoub, I. (2012). Robotic surgery: a review on recent advances in surgical robotic systems. *Florida Conference on Recent Advances in Robotics*, 2012.

17. Mathur, S., & Sutton, J. (2017, July 01). Personalized medicine could transform healthcare (review). Retrieved May 01, 2021, from https://www.spandidos-publications.com /10.3892/br.2017.922?text=fulltext

6 Crop Variety Selection to Enhance the Yield Rate of Crops by Applying Machine Learning Methods

S. Iniyan, R. Jebakumar, Rishav Raj
and Rituparna Singh

CONTENTS

DOI: 10.1201/9781003132110-6

6.1 INTRODUCTION

The main goal for agriculture is the maximum production of crops on a limited land size. If the problem that is associated with crop production were determined then it would be much easier for an individual to grow the crop with maximum yield. Selection of the correct crop for a particular land can be useful for farmers in order to increase crop production and maximize their profit.

If we are successful in using fewer resources—either money, land or fertilizers—while producing maximum yield, then the goal of agricultural planning is reached, which can be done with the help of various machine learning and artificial intelligence techniques. During unfavourable conditions, there is a great need to wisely select a particular type of crop to increase the crop yield rate. It can be achieved using various strategies which can be either manual or AI-based, but the major drawback of the manual method is labour cost and more time. Also, due to certain failures, backtracking is not possible. We will be taking into consideration various parameters like amount of rainfall, humidity, quality of seed, land quality and terrain/grassland and will apply univariate and bivariate analysis on the features to get a clear idea of how features are interdependent and affect yield rate.

The crop selection mainly depends on favourable and unfavourable conditions. Till now various studies have been carried out in this field to improve agricultural planning with the ultimate goal of getting maximum yield.

Crop production is largely influenced by various climatic as well as geographic conditions like rivers, terrain, grassland, humidity, temperature and amount of rain. The type of soil can be sandy, clayey, saline, etc. and have a composition of elements like Cu, K, P, N, Mn, Fe, Ca and pH value of carbon. All of these parameters and certain new parameters like hours needed and the farmer's own willingness to promote a particular crop in a region play important roles. So, all these can be broadly divided into two categories: traditional and machine learning algorithms.

6.1.1 ARTIFICIAL NEURAL NETWORK (ANN)

An artificial neural network is an interconnection between different units that are recognised as weighted processing units. In the processing unit, input can be given and output as well. The input is given from the previous processing units and the output is for other processing units. In general, the topological algorithms used are multi-layered perceptron and backpropagation [1]. We can use an artificial neural network at the place where the number of attributes is less.

6.1.2 DECISION TREE

In a decision tree, the root node, which is the first node, holds all the sample spaces present for the model. Further, it is subdivided into sub-sample spaces that can be easily formulated by a simple model [2]. The parent nodes are divided into different child nodes. And this division can take place recursively. The division can take place according to the condition given by the input values. The splitting can be according to the impurity measures and node size. There are different algorithms that can be used for making a decision tree such as CART [3], M5-Prime and Prime [2]. M5-Prime is another version of M5 that can be used in order to deal with missing values and enumerated attributes. M5 is more smooth and good as compared to the CART algorithm.

6.1.3 RANDOM FOREST

RF algorithm was first created by Tin Kam Ho with the help of the random subspace method. Random forest is an ensemble learning method [4] used for different purposes like classification, regression, etc. These various sub-parts are created with random sub-sampled features. It can be used for high-dimension inputs. In random forest, the output is taken as an average of the values given by different individual trees.

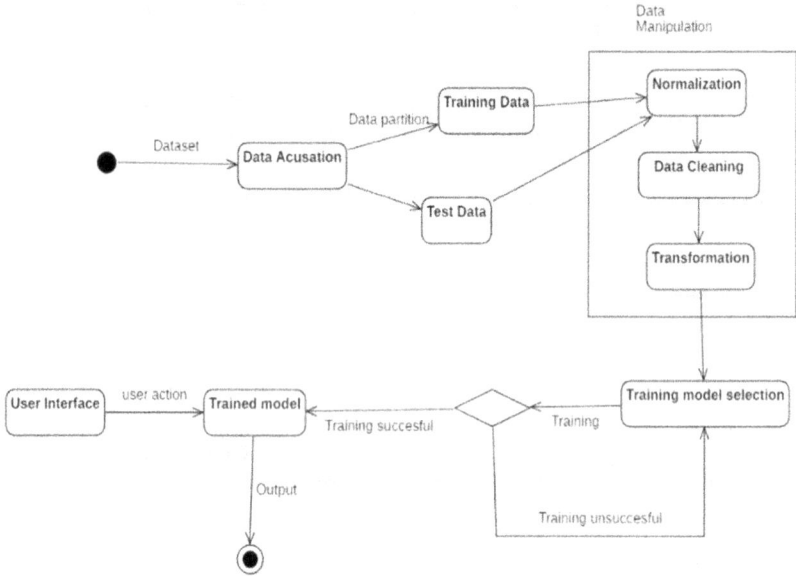

FIGURE 6.1 System architecture.

6.1.4 SYSTEM ARCHITECTURE

The approach simply follows an architectural diagram of crop variety selection to enhance the yield rate of crops by applying machine learning methods (Figure 6.1).

In this architecture diagram, we can see how the system works in crop variety selection. First, input is given which means a set of datasets is provided to us for further classification. After that, data acquisition is split into two parts which are testing data and training dataset, where testing data involvement is 30% and training data involvement is 70%. Training data will be labelled data which is predefined through which prediction will occur and testing data measures how accurate data is and how efficiently it is working. After training and testing, we come to the data manipulation part, where three processes are shown, which are normalisation, data cleaning and transformation. In this step of data manipulation, first data will be analysed where an objective variable decision is made and determination of high cardinality helps in visualisation in scatterplots which is a superior system. Secondly, in data cleaning, high cardinality factors are cleaned. And in transformation, erasing of objective variables has taken place from the whole collected information and changed straight out factors in a model framework with one-hot encoding. This is once in a while the interest for specific calculations to process the information in a scanty framework group. I ascribed the missing qualities inside the information to 0. I scaled the persistent factors by utilising the min-max standardisation which changes esteems onto a scale from 0 to 1 to square factors on various scales vigorously affecting the coefficients.

After the data manipulation step, training of model selection is done. We apportioned the pre-handled information into the preparation and test informational index. Data partitioning is a classification in supervised machine learning which is used to separate pre-defined classes of data. This is typically used in splitting the data into multiple chunks. Data partition can be used in obtaining both training and testing datasets. Now our training is successful then we will be moving to a trained model to get our desired output but if training is unsuccessful then we need to repeat training model selection. Now in evaluation, we scored the classifier on inconspicuous test information and determined the R-squared data for both the preparation and test information regarding how the output would be obtained. Our output will be displayed on the interface which can be an Android application or a Windows-based application.

6.1.4.1   Data Synthesis

Crop variety selection depends on various factors like production of data from taking trials on fields, analysing sensors and representation of different types of farmers' and consumers' participation. Data synthesis helps in producing new information about decision-making by combining with previous and new data (Figure 6.2).

Data synthesis plays a part in the selection of crops to improve accuracy by conducting multiple assessments. The types of data that are required to evaluate crop variety selection are agronomic performance data, environment data and food status and consumer-preference details.

6.1.4.1.1   Agronomic Performance Data

Data are taken by making trials on fields by various classifications: 1) internationally public breeding programmes, 2) hidden programmes with trading seed companies and 3) national-level agriculture research. Basically, there are two categories of trials: breed and official trials, which release the set of data on which the classification

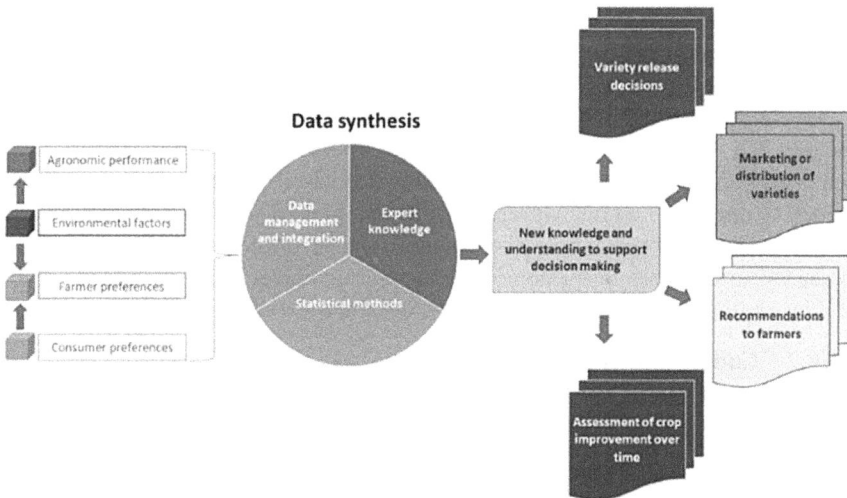

FIGURE 6.2   Various factors and processes involved in data synthesis.

will be performed. Collected data from trials involves the location of the trial, date and observation of the trial.

6.1.4.1.2   Environmental Data

Breaking down the phenotypic reaction of genotypes to the testing environment is a principal stage to describe the surroundings. The climate is the main cause of yield changeability in plant-rearing preliminaries. Thus, ecological data are needed to portray the preliminary area and to comprehend its impact on the presentation of tried genotypes in that defined area. This is realised for utilisation of ecological information as model covariates dissecting multi-area preliminary information improve the degree of exactness in the expectation of genotypic execution.

Ecological information can be gathered at preliminary sites directly. Be that as it may, regardless of whether natural information was not gathered during preliminaries, geolocating preliminary destinations permits enhancing the dataset with ecological information. Adding ecological information to legacy preliminary information permits examinations among preliminaries led at different areas. A few sorts of ecological information are increasingly accessible through open and public storehouses. For example, information-based precipitation, temperature, elevations and soils are transparently and unreservedly accessible from open and public databases like the Climate Hazards group's Infrared Precipitation with Stations (CHIRPS) dataset.

6.1.4.1.3   Food Quality and Consumer Preference Data

Sensor-based and health assessments have gotten more attention in recent years, countering the tight focal point of harvest improvement on yield, sickness obstruction and consistency. As of now, shopper markets are evolving, with customers looking for extra item characteristics such as nutritional and sensorial attributes. Food status includes paired levelheaded and emotional analyses, including estimations of substance and surface, along with sensor-based investigations. Tactile assessment is officially characterised as a scientific rule used to inspire, estimate, investigate and between pert responses to those attributes of food varieties and materials as they sense by the feelings of sight, aroma, flavour, touch and sound.

Agronomic execution, nourishment quality and inclination data are quite costly and complex to procure and oversee. Compared to this, climate and topsoil information is progressively accessible at remarkably decreased expenses. Extra exertion is needed to upgrade the effectiveness of information used in the assessment of yield varieties. The larger accessibility of climate and topsoil information can inspire and increment information utilisation, repurposing inheritance crops assortment tested data by joining ecological information to extricate fresh experiences.

6.1.4.2   Coding and Testing

The analysis in this chapter is performed using random forest and a decision tree and involves the following software.

6.1.4.2.1   Programming Environment

We have used Jupyter Notebook, an open-source web app that is utilised to generate and share files containing codes, statistics and equations.

6.1.4.2.2   Programming Language

With the assistance of different Python libraries, we have fostered this task. A portion of the essential libraries, for example, NumPy, Matplotlib, Seaborn and Pandas, is utilised for essential tasks and AI libraries like Scikit-learn are used for the execution of different calculations.

6.1.4.2.3   Exploratory Visualisation

Throughout this progression, we played out some distinct investigating and decided on the objective variable. We additionally found what number of classes were in the objective and a determination of other conceivably tricky (high cardinality) factors. I likewise visualised the objective variable in a scatterplot which is a superior system for understanding the circulation of the information to aid parameter tuning.

6.1.4.2.4   Graphic User Interface

We have made a GUI with help of the Tkinter GUI toolkit. Tkinter naming is done by an interface of Tk, which is a standard Py interface, connected with the Tkinter GUI toolkit. It includes the standard Windows, Mac OS and Linux. This GUI will show the output as per the input given. As soon as input is given a graphical interface comes on screen with expected output and the Jupyter platform is used for executing the GUI.

6.1.4.2.5   Database

A dataset is taken to get accurate results by checking every dataset with input given, and whatever the input matches with, that is our result. Our dataset is a predefined set of models which is labelled. The database is managed in a group in a way that it can simply access, manage and update. SQL is mostly used when we are handling the database which is helpful in records by inserting, deleting or updating the previous record. A database is constructed which contains crop variety selection data and total number of data consisting of 242,361 rows and seven different columns along with 3,730 null values in column "production".

6.1.4.2.6   Testing

Testing was done by a scoring classifier on inconspicuous test information and it determined the R-squared data for both the preparation and test information regarding the output. And after successful testing output will be shown in the form of a GUI interface.

6.2   LITERATURE SURVEY

In a conference chapter on "Crop Selection Method to Maximize Crop Yield Rate Using Machine Learning Technique", a CSM algorithm predicts the yield rate of crops based on suitable conditions prior and produces a series of crops with greater yield rate [5]. CSM retrieves all crops to be produces at a given duration of time. If the yield rate is favourable then crops can be taken from crop series or sequences. The time that's given after the harvesting time of crops is the time stamp for upcoming crop selection. Hence multiple crop sequences with varying yield rates are produced.

So, the crop sequence has the highest or more net yield rate as compared to another crop taken for crop sequencing.

According to Kaur [6], machine learning is a field of AI that has a broad range of use in various fields like weather monitoring/forecasting, pattern recognition, gaming etc. In agriculture also we can incorporate this technology. Finding disease types in crops, the prediction of crop yield and the use of smart systems like smart irrigation systems are some of the fields where machine learning is of great help if applied properly. The feed-forward backpropagation ANN can be used for a better crop yield rate of crops.

Paras et al. [7] have given a weather forecasting model that is feature-based. RNN, a recurrent neural network which is a variant of an artificial neural network, is used in weather prediction.

According to Kumar et al. [8], agriculture in India mostly depends upon monsoon rainfall.

In Raorane and Kulkarni [9], relationship analysis of crop and climate is carried out with the help of older statistics of production for major crops like groundnut, sugarcane, rice and wheat and aggregate foods like grain, pulses and oilseed to study and understand the correlation between crop and climatic condition. It provides information on monsoon rainfall influence and also some possible predictors of crop production. Various data mining techniques and older data on crop yield are helpful to get data.

In Navarro-Hell [10], a machine learning DSS is presented by Navarro-Hell to predict the requirements for one week of irrigation using prediction mechanisms which include ANFIS and PSLR. Patil et al. presented a crop disease prediction system.

Khosla et al. [11] used a model to predict crop yield support vector regression. And rainfall is predicted using MANN and then depending upon rainfall amount and other parameters like moisture, temperature rainfall and atmospheric pressure. It also indicates the best time for sowing and harvesting a certain crop.

In Priya et al. [12], a naïve Bayes classification technique suitable for crops such as rice, cotton, maize and chilli in Visakhapatnam is carried out for weather parameters like rainfall, soil moisture, etc.

In Kumar et al. [13], a crop selection method is used to increase crop yield rate and it suggests crop sequence planted over a year to gain maximum yield. Classification of crops is done into different categories depending on growing time: (1) seasonal, (2) whole year, (3) short-duration and (4) long-duration. The crop selection is depending on soil, weather, kind of crop and also water density factors. After crop selection, a crop sequencing mechanism is carried out which gives better yield based upon plantation day, crop, predicted yield and time of sowing.

6.3   DATA PREPROCESSING AND PRELIMINARY ANALYSIS

6.3.1   META INFORMATION

This data consists of district-wise, crop-wise, season-wise and year-wise data on crop covered areas and production. This data can be used for analysis and study of crop production and crop selection algorithms of different states/districts/countries. There is dependence on climatic factors for agricultural yield of crops, crop growing patterns and diversification. The features are used for analysis of past year crop production based on several climatic and soil parameters. Other features like Production_Per_Unit_Area, Rainfall and Quality of Soil can be further added to this dataset for regional analysis shown in Figures 6.3–6.9.

6.3.2 DATA DESCRIPTION

1. Size of data—246,091 rows and 7 columns
2. Dimensionality—7
3. Feature description (attributes)—State_Name, District_Name, Crop_Year, Season, Crop, Area, Production
4. Nominal (discrete)—State, District, Crop_Year, Season, Crop
5. Interval (continuous)—Area, Production
6. Independent features—State_Name, District_Name, Crop_Year, Season, Crop, Area
7. Dependent feature—Production

6.3.3 DATA QUALITY

1. None—No such extraneous object is shown that would modify the original value
2. Outliers—Outliers are observed in the box plot as explained later in the documentation
3. Missing values—There are 3,730 missing values in the Production column and no other columns have missing values
4. Duplicate data—No duplicate rows are present in the dataset

6.3.4 DATA PREPROCESSING

It is the process by which raw data is transform into a useful facts which is available for the user.

6.3.4.1 Importing Libraries and Dataset

```
In [1]: import pandas as pd
        import numpy as np
        import matplotlib.pyplot as plt
        %matplotlib inline
        import seaborn as sns

In [2]: df = pd.read_csv('crop_production.csv')

In [3]: df.head()

Out[3]:
```

	State_Name	District_Name	Crop_Year	Season	Crop	Area	Production
0	Andaman and Nicobar Islands	NICOBARS	2000	Kharif	Arecanut	1254.0	2000.0
1	Andaman and Nicobar Islands	NICOBARS	2000	Kharif	Other Kharif pulses	2.0	1.0
2	Andaman and Nicobar Islands	NICOBARS	2000	Kharif	Rice	102.0	321.0
3	Andaman and Nicobar Islands	NICOBARS	2000	Whole Year	Banana	176.0	641.0
4	Andaman and Nicobar Islands	NICOBARS	2000	Whole Year	Cashewnut	720.0	165.0

FIGURE 6.3 Crop dataset is imported.

6.3.4.2   Determining the Size of the Dataset

```
In [5]: df.shape
Out[5]: (246091, 7)
```

FIGURE 6.4   Shape of dataset.

6.3.4.3   Determining Features of the Dataset

```
In [4]: df.columns
Out[4]: Index(['State_Name', 'District_Name', 'Crop_Year', 'Season', 'Crop', 'Area',
               'Production'],
              dtype='object')
```

FIGURE 6.5   Column names.

6.3.5   DATA EXPLORATION

This step is used to analyze and explore the data to dig into more.

6.3.5.1   Extracting Missing Values from the Dataset

```
In [6]: df.isnull().sum()
Out[6]: State_Name         0
        District_Name      0
        Crop_Year          0
        Season             0
        Crop               0
        Area               0
        Production      3730
        dtype: int64
```

FIGURE 6.6   Missing values.

6.3.5.2   Removing Duplicates

```
In [7]: data = df.dropna()
        print(data.shape)
        test = df[~df['Production'].notna()].drop('Production', axis=1)
        print(test.shape)

        (242361, 7)
        (3730, 6)
```

FIGURE 6.7   Removing duplicates.

6.3.5.3 Finding the Measure of Central Tendency by Using the Describe() Function

```
In [8]: df.describe(include='all')
Out[8]:
```

	State_Name	District_Name	Crop_Year	Season	Crop	Area	Production
count	246091	246091	246091.000000	246091	246091	2.460910e+05	2.423610e+05
unique	33	646	NaN	6	124	NaN	NaN
top	Uttar Pradesh	BIJAPUR	NaN	Kharif	Rice	NaN	NaN
freq	33306	945	NaN	95951	15104	NaN	NaN
mean	NaN	NaN	2005.643018	NaN	NaN	1.200282e+04	5.825034e+05
std	NaN	NaN	4.952164	NaN	NaN	5.052340e+04	1.706581e+07
min	NaN	NaN	1997.000000	NaN	NaN	4.000000e-02	0.000000e+00
25%	NaN	NaN	2002.000000	NaN	NaN	8.000000e+01	8.800000e+01
50%	NaN	NaN	2006.000000	NaN	NaN	5.820000e+02	7.290000e+02
75%	NaN	NaN	2010.000000	NaN	NaN	4.392000e+03	7.023000e+03
max	NaN	NaN	2015.000000	NaN	NaN	8.580100e+06	1.250800e+09

FIGURE 6.8 Describing the dataset.

6.3.5.4 Viewing the Datatypes of All Features

```
In [12]: data.dtypes
Out[12]: State_Name        object
         District_Name     object
         Crop_Year         int64
         Season            object
         Crop              object
         Area              float64
         Production        float64
         dtype: object

In [13]: data.groupby('Season')['Production'].sum()
Out[13]: Season
         Autumn          6.441377e+07
         Kharif          4.029970e+09
         Rabi            2.051688e+09
         Summer          1.706579e+08
         Whole Year      1.344248e+11
         Winter          4.345498e+08
         Name: Production, dtype: float64
```

FIGURE 6.9 Datatypes of dataset.

6.3.6 BI-VARIATE ANALYSIS

6.3.6.1 Co-Relation between Crop Year and Production

```
In [9]: sns.lineplot(data["Crop_Year"],data["Production"])

         C:\Users\Hp\anaconda3\lib\site-packages\seaborn\_decorators.py:36: FutureWarning: Pass the following variables
         as keyword args: x, y. From version 0.12, the only valid positional argument will be `data`, and passing
         other arguments without an explicit key word will result in an error or misinterpretation.
           warnings.warn(

Out[9]: <AxesSubplot:xlabel='Crop_Year', ylabel='Production'>
```

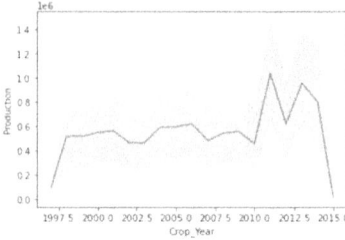

FIGURE 6.10   Crop year versus production.

From the above line-plot, we can see that the crop production highly increased during the years 2010–2015. The reason may be due to the involvement of several scientific and modern agricultural techniques in the farming sector as well as an increase in the data record and high data collection.

6.3.6.2 Co-Relation between Season and Production

From the below plot we see that 95.2% of crops are grown the whole year followed by the Kharif season. The autumn season has the lowest crop production rate.

```
In [15]: tot = df['Production'].sum()

In [17]: data.groupby('Season')['Production'].sum()*100/tot

Out[17]: Season
         Autumn            0.045627
         Kharif            2.854569
         Rabi              1.453282
         Summer            0.120883
         Whole Year       95.217832
         Winter            0.307807
         Name: Production, dtype: float64
```

FIGURE 6.11   Season versus production (tabular).

Each type of crop requires a different area and season parameter so the analysis of the top crop is carried out here.

From Figure 6.13 we observe that the top five produced crops are:

```
In [11]: sns.barplot(data["Season"],data["Production"])

         C:\Users\Hp\anaconda3\lib\site-packages\seaborn\_decorators.py:36: FutureWarning: Pass the following variables
         as keyword args: x, y. From version 0.12, the only valid positional argument will be `data`, and passing
         other arguments without an explicit key word will result in an error or misinterpretation.
           warnings.warn(

Out[11]: <AxesSubplot:xlabel='Season', ylabel='Production'>
```

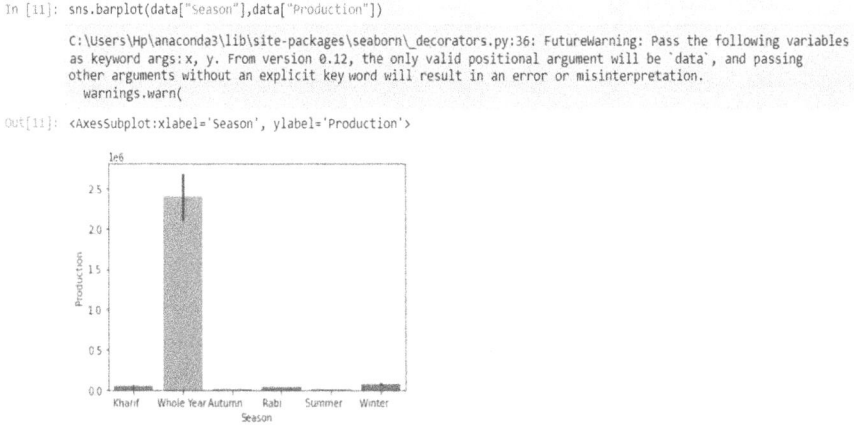

FIGURE 6.12   Season versus production (graphical).

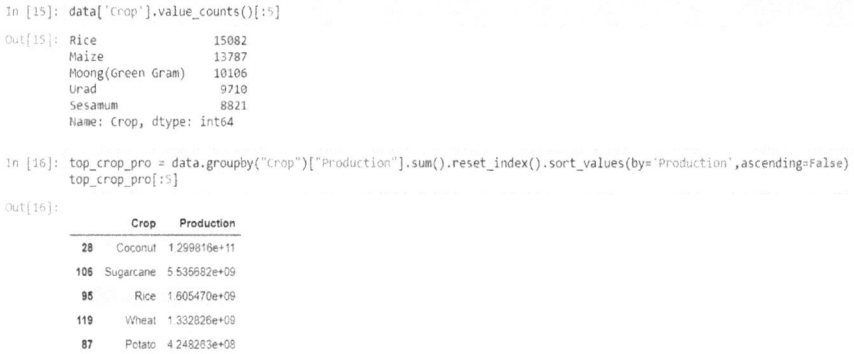

```
In [15]: data['Crop'].value_counts()[:5]

Out[15]: Rice                   15082
         Maize                  13787
         Moong(Green Gram)      10106
         Urad                    9710
         Sesamum                 8821
         Name: Crop, dtype: int64

In [16]: top_crop_pro = data.groupby("Crop")["Production"].sum().reset_index().sort_values(by='Production',ascending=False)
         top_crop_pro[:5]

Out[16]:
```

	Crop	Production
28	Coconut	1.299816e+11
106	Sugarcane	5.535682e+09
95	Rice	1.605470e+09
119	Wheat	1.332826e+09
87	Potato	4.248263e+08

FIGURE 6.13   List of top crops.

1. Coconut
2. Sugarcane
3. Rice
4. Wheat
5. Potato

There are some of the crops which are not at all produced. They are:

Based on the kind of crops and to do a common analysis of similar types of crops, the crops are grouped into categories. For example, "Rice", "Maize", "Wheat", "Barley", "Varagu", "Other cereals and millets", "Ragi", "Small millets", "Bajra" and "Jowar" are grouped as cereals. "Moong", "Urad", "Arhar/Tur", "Peas and beans", "Masoor", "Other Kharif pulses", "Other misc. pulses", "Ricebean (nagadal)", "Rajmash," "Blackgram", "Korra", "Cowpea (Lobia)", "Other Rabi pulses", "Other Kharif pulses" and "Peas and beans (pulses)" are grouped as pulses.

Most Produced Crop

```
In [53]: temp = data.groupby('Crop')['Production'].sum().reset_index().sort_values(by='Production', ascending=False)
         sns.barplot(temp['Crop'].head(),temp['Production'].head())

         C:\Users\Hp\anaconda3\lib\site-packages\seaborn\_decorators.py:36: FutureWarning: Pass the following variables
         as keyword args: x, y. From version 0.12, the only valid positional argument will be `data`, and passing
         other arguments without an explicit key word will result in an error or misinterpretation.
           warnings.warn(
```

Out[53]: <AxesSubplot:xlabel='Crop', ylabel='Production'>

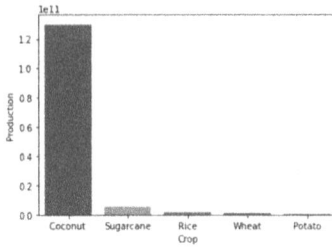

FIGURE 6.14 Most produced crop (graphical).

None Produced Crop

In [54]: temp[temp['Production']==0].reset_index(drop=True)

Out[54]:

	Crop	Production
0	other fibres	0.0
1	Yam	0.0
2	Water Melon	0.0
3	Ash Gourd	0.0
4	Beet Root	0.0
5	Plums	0.0
6	Ber	0.0
7	Snak Guard	0.0
8	Ribed Guard	0.0
9	Pump Kin	0.0
10	Peas (vegetable)	0.0
11	Pear	0.0
12	Peach	0.0
13	Other Dry Fruit	0.0
14	Other Citrus Fruit	0.0
15	Cucumber	0.0
16	Litchi	0.0
17	Lab-Lab	0.0
18	Apple	0.0

FIGURE 6.15 Non-produced crops.

6.3.7   DATA VISUALISATION

Each type of crop requires different area and season parameters so the analysis of the top crops is carried out here.

6.3.7.1   Rice

Rice production mostly depends on area, state and season.

```
In [58]: data.head()
Out[58]:
```

	State_Name	District_Name	Crop_Year	Season	Crop	Area	Production	cat_crop
0	Andaman and Nicobar Islands	NICOBARS	2000	Kharif	Arecanut	1254 0	2000.0	Nuts
1	Andaman and Nicobar Islands	NICOBARS	2000	Kharif	Other Kharif pulses	2 0	1 0	Pulses
2	Andaman and Nicobar Islands	NICOBARS	2000	Kharif	Rice	102 0	321.0	Cereal
3	Andaman and Nicobar Islands	NICOBARS	2000	Whole Year	Banana	176.0	641 0	Fruits
4	Andaman and Nicobar Islands	NICOBARS	2000	Whole Year	Cashewnut	720 0	165 0	Nuts

```
In [59]: data["cat_crop"].value_counts()
Out[59]: Cereal            62607
         Pulses            33405
         Oilseeds          33375
         Species           21631
         Vegetables        21559
         Beans             17926
         Nuts              11472
         Sugarcane          7827
         fibres             7602
         Fruits             6153
         Commercial         2637
         Fertile Plant      2183
         Paddy               479
         Oilseeds total      426
         Pulses total        266
         Total foodgrain     188
         Tea                  62
         Natural Polymer      29
         Other                27
         Coffee                6
         Name: cat_crop, dtype: int64
```

FIGURE 6.16   Kinds of crops.

6.3.7.2   Coconut

- Coconut production does not depend on season.
- Coconut production is directly proportional to area.
- The production is highest in Kerala.
- The production increases every year.

6.3.7.3   Sugarcane

- Sugarcane production is high in some states only.
- Sugarcane production is directly proportional to area.

The datatypes are:

- State _ Name : object
- District _ Name : object

- Crop _ Year : integer
- Season : object
- Crop : object
- Area : float
- Production : float

6.4 CROP SELECTION METHOD

In our system, we are making use of classification algorithms to improve crop yields.

The algorithms may vary depending on the accuracy we will get. The algorithms mostly include naive Bayes, decision trees, random forest classifier, ensemble models and advanced ML algorithms like artificial neural networks and backpropagation algorithms.

The various stages of predictive modelling will include:

1. Defining the problem statement.
2. Generation of unbiased hypothesis.
3. Data extraction/collection.
4. Data exploration and transformation.
5. Predictive modelling.
6. Model deployment/implementation.

The metrics we will be using are accuracy, TPR, TNR, FPR, FNR, recall and precision, AUC-ROC metric and log loss. The Python libraries Keras, Scikit-learn, Matplotlib, Numpy, Tensorflow and Pandas will be used.

6.5 OBJECTIVE OF THE PROJECT

1. The purpose of incorporating machine learning in the field of crop yield prediction is to minimise the cost and resources including labour cost, transportation cost, pesticides and fertiliser cost and others.
2. The yield can be maximised to a large extent if we are having a prediction of the best-suited crop in a particular region based on several parameters and previous data using predictive modelling.
3. Land utilisation and quality of crops can be improved by self-learning algorithms so that they can predict what needs to be done under what circumstances.

6.6 SCOPE OF THE PROJECT

Our model will be available as open-source software, so that it can be accessed and used by everyone who needs it. It will not be limited to any community and will be updated according to the needs of the people. Updates can be given via Android application update or software update.

6.7   MODULE DESCRIPTION

6.7.1   Exploratory Data Analysis

Throughout this progression, we played out some distinct investigations and decided on the objective variable. We additionally found what number of classes were in the objective and a determination of other conceivably tricky (high cardinality) factors. I likewise visualised the objective variable in a scatterplot which is a superior system for understanding the circulation of the information to aid parameter tuning.

6.7.2   Data Cleaning

We dropped those high cardinality factors during this procedure as an antecedent to the pre-handling step.

6.7.3   Preprocessing and Transformation

We erased the objective variable from the whole informational collection and changed the straight-out factor into a model framework with one-hot encoding. This is once in a while the interest for specific calculations to process the information in a scanty framework group. I ascribed the missing qualities inside the information to 0. I scaled the persistent factors by utilising the min-max standardisation which changes esteems onto a scale from 0 to 1 to square factors on various scales vigorously affecting the coefficients.

6.7.4   Data Training Model

6.7.4.1   Data Partition

We apportioned the pre-handled information into the preparation and test informational index. Data partitioning is a classification in supervised machine learning which is used to separate pre-defined classes of data. This is typically used in splitting the data into multiple chunks. Data partition can be used in obtaining both training and testing datasets.

6.7.5   Testing and Evaluation Model

6.7.5.1   Evaluation

We scored the classifier on inconspicuous test information and determined that the R-squared data for both the preparation and test information regarding the output would be obtained.

6.7.6   Output Model

The output will be displayed on the interface which can be an Android application or a Windows-based application.

6.8 ALGORITHMS/METHODOLOGY

6.8.1 DECISION TREE

A decision tree uses a tree model which consists of left and right sub-trees in which possible outcomes including probability, cost of resources and utilities are predicted. It uses impurity measures to check for the given criteria and whichever feature gives the most suitable outcome is chosen as a node to split. It consists of conditional flow control mechanisms.

6.8.1.1 Parameters on Which Decision Tree Predicts Outcome

There are two major concepts involved in this—information gain and entropy.

6.8.1.2 Entropy

It measures how randomly a system performs. It is the expected count of bits that are required for encoding a random class member of given sample space S.

Entropy is given by the below formula:

$$\text{Entropy } E\left(\text{Sample}\right) = - \bullet p\left(\text{feature}\right) * \log 2\left(p\left(\text{feature}\right)\right)$$

6.8.1.3 Information Gain

It is the measure of the decrease in entropy of a system due to the splitting of a class. The tree is presented using the outcomes.

6.8.2 RANDOM FOREST

Random forest (RF) consists of n DT having a different set of parameters and training on a different dataset. Suppose 100 DTs are there in a random forest bag. Since the parameters and training dataset are different the prediction which we will get from each and every D-tree will vary a lot. Suppose all these 100 trees are trained on a respective subset of data. So to take a final decision on a particular test data of a certain decision tree we go by the process of voting. The outcome predicted by the majority of trees is selected as a feature to split. The outcome of a D-tree varies from one tree to another as each and every feature has different values of entropy and information gain. So, we use RFs to get the most common prediction and the feature corresponding to it is selected starting from the root node to the leaf node.

RF is reliable and stable compared to one single D-tree. It is similar to having a poll of all ministers before taking any decision rather than a single decision taken by the prime minister.

In Figure 6.16 it is shown that a single instance has been classed with n D-tree and the final output is generated by voting from all n trees. In ML, RFs are also known as ensemble/bagging models.

RF is a supervised learning method which can be used for both classification and regression tasks. It is widely used because it is a stable and simple ML algorithm. RF has a wide range of applications in various fields such as pattern recognising, NLP and handwritten text classification. It makes use of bagging and boosting algorithms for the selection of the most suitable features and an equal split of features for each and every D-tree.

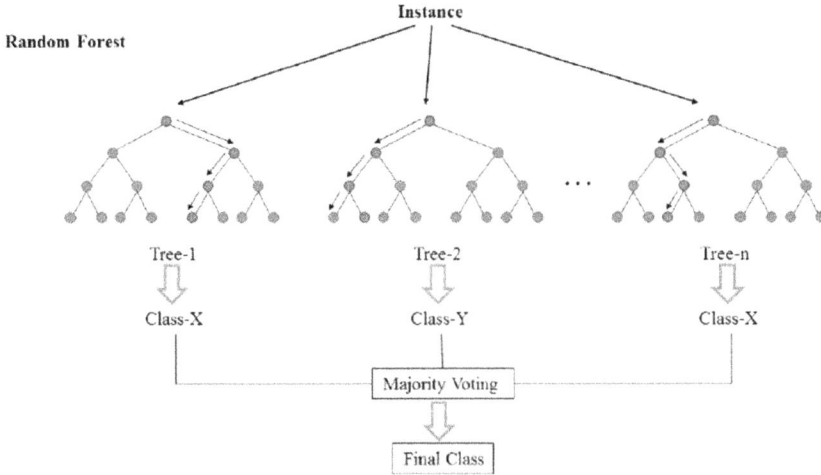

FIGURE 6.17   Random forest flow diagram.

A random dataset is created using bagging and boosting algorithms. It selects k features (columns) and one feature (row), and the rest (n-k) and (m-l) features are used for other datasets where n and m are columns and rows of the original dataset.

6.8.2.1   Implementation of Random Forest

Model 2 - Random Forest Classifier

```
In [93]: from sklearn.ensemble import RandomForestClassifier
         from sklearn.metrics import roc_auc_score
         sample_leaf_options = [1,2,3,4,5,10,20]

         for leaf_size in sample_leaf_options :
             model = RandomForestClassifier(n_estimators = 200, n_jobs = -1,random_state =50, min_samples_leaf = leaf_size)
             model.fit(train_x,train_y)
             print("\n Leaf size :", leaf_size)
             print ("AUC - ROC : ", accuracy_score(train_y,model.predict(train_x)))


         <ipython-input-93-cb50ca010534>:8: DataConversionWarning: A column-vector y was passed when a 1d array was
         expected. Please change the shape of y to (n_samples,), for example using ravel().
           model.fit(train_x,train_y)

          Leaf size : 1
         AUC - ROC :  1.0

         <ipython-input-93-cb50ca010534>:8: DataConversionWarning: A column-vector y was passed when a 1d array was
         expected. Please change the shape of y to (n_samples,), for example using ravel().
           model.fit(train_x,train_y)

          Leaf size : 2
         AUC - ROC :  0.9803030303030303

         <ipython-input-93-cb50ca010534>:8: DataConversionWarning: A column-vector y was passed when a 1d array was
         expected. Please change the shape of y to (n_samples,), for example using ravel().
           model.fit(train_x,train_y)

          Leaf size : 3
         AUC - ROC :  0.9359848484848485

         <ipython-input-93-cb50ca010534>:8: DataConversionWarning: A column-vector y was passed when a 1d array was
         expected. Please change the shape of y to (n_samples,), for example using ravel().
           model.fit(train_x,train_y)
```

FIGURE 6.18   Output of random forest algorithm.

6.8.3   K-Nearest Neighbor

It falls in the class of supervised learning that is useful in rectifying issues of classification and regression. Generally, it is preferred for predictive classification.

6.8.3.1   Two Properties of KNN

1. Lazy learning algorithm.

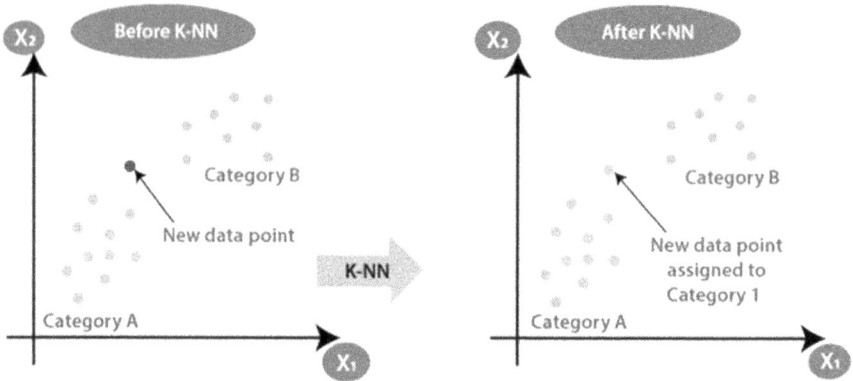

FIGURE 6.19   Need for KNN.

As its name says it is lazy because it does not have a proper standardised phase of training so when classification is to be performed it utilises complete given data to train.

2. Non-parametric learning algorithm.

It is not parametric as assumptions are not made for underlying data.

6.8.3.2   Need for KNN

We need KNN in case a new data point is there and there are two categories, suppose category A and B, but we do not know to which category this new data point should be placed, so here KNN helps to identify to which category data points belong. See the diagram given in Figure 6.19.

6.8.3.2.1   Steps of Algorithm

```
step 1: selection of number k from neighbours.
step 2: find out Euclidean distance of K.
step 3: take step2 value then mark the K nearest
    neighbour.
```

step 4: find out the number of data points in all
   categories.
step 5: analyse the maximum number of neighbours and
   then categorise each data point.
step 6: we get our model ready.

Step 1, where k = 5
Step 2: data point is categorised.

6.8.3.3   Implementation of KNN Algorithm

KNN Algorithm mentioned below and it has KNN Classifier with the output which is shown in Figure 6.20.

Model 3 - KNN Classifier

```
In [101]: from sklearn.neighbors import KNeighborsClassifier as KNN

          reg = KNN(n_neighbors = 5)
          reg.fit(train_x, train_y)
          train_predict = reg.predict(train_x)
          k = accuracy_score(train_y, train_predict)
          print('Train KNN Accuracy score : ',k)

          <ipython-input-101-04a0acd8c16c>:4: DataConversionWarning: A column-vector y was passed when
          a 1d array was expected. Please change the shape of y to (n_samples, ), for example using ravel().
            reg.fit(train_x, train_y)

          Train KNN Accuracy score :  0.4683080808080808

In [102]: valid_predict = reg.predict(valid_x)
          k1 = accuracy_score(valid_y, valid_predict)
          print('Validation KNN Accuracy score : ',k1)

          Validation KNN Accuracy score :  0.2474747474747475

In [103]: test_predict = reg.predict(test_x)
          k2 = accuracy_score(test_y, test_predict)
          print('Test KNN Accuracy score : ',k2)

          Test KNN Accuracy score :  0.2568659127625202

In [104]: print('Training KNN accuracy score:', k)
          print('Validation KNN accuracy score:', k1)
          print('Testing KNN accuracy score:', k2)

          Training KNN accuracy score: 0.4683080808080808
          Validation KNN accuracy score: 0.2474747474747475
          Testing KNN accuracy score: 0.2568659127625202

In [105]: test_predict[:5],test_y[:5]

Out[105]: (array(['Horse-gram', 'Sweet potato', 'Sunflower', 'Jowar', 'Cashewnut'],
```

FIGURE 6.20   Output of KNN algorithm.

6.8.4   LOGISTIC REGRESSION

It falls in the class of supervised learning that is useful in predicting category-wise dependent variables from independent variables.

It makes predictions for dependent numerals' output and provides results in binary a value, either 0 or 1, true or false, and so on. But most of the time it delivers value in a statistical manner which is in the range of 0 and 1.

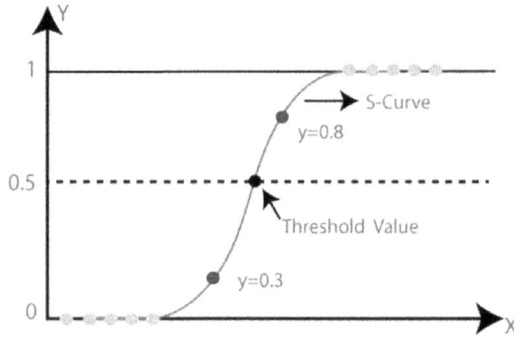

FIGURE 6.21   S-curved graph.

It can be seen that logistic regression is the same as linear regression but using techniques that are different. Logistic regression helps in classification and linear helps in regression problems.

There is no purpose of regression to fit a line; instead, we use an S-shaped logistic function which gives two outputs in between 0 and 1.

It is a noteworthy ML algorithm as it can give probability and can-do classification of new data with the help of discrete data and also classifies different types of data.

These equations are acquired by linear regression:

We know the straight-line equation:

$$y = b_0 + b_1 x_1 + b_2 x_2 + b_3 x_3 + \cdots + b_n x_n$$

Y tends for 0 in logistic:

$$\frac{y}{1-y}; 0 \text{ for } y = 0, \text{ and infinity for } y = 1$$

And we need in the range of − infinity to + infinity:

$$\log\left[\frac{y}{1-y}\right] = b_0 + b_1 x_1 + b_2 x_2 + b_3 x_3 + \cdots + b_n x_n$$

6.8.4.1   Logistic Sigmoid Function

It helps in mapping the predicted value to the probability of data in range 0 and 1 and its range should not exceed the given limit; then afterward it forms a structure of s which is known as sigmoid function. Threshold value comes into the picture in this case that helps in defining probabilities in the range of 0 and 1.

- Category is important in this case.
- Multi-colinearity should not be there.

6.8.4.2   Implementation of Logistic Regression Algorithm

Logistic regression algorithm mentioned below.

```
In [88]:  from sklearn.linear_model import LogisticRegression as LogReg
          from sklearn.metrics import f1_score

In [89]:  logreg = LogReg()
          logreg.fit(train_x, train_y)

          C:\Users\Hp\anaconda3\lib\site-packages\sklearn\utils\validation.py:72: DataConversionWarning: A column-vector
          y was passed when a 1d array was expected. Please change the shape of y to (n_samples, ), for example using ravel().
            return f(**kwargs)
          C:\Users\Hp\anaconda3\lib\site-packages\sklearn\linear_model\_logistic.py:762: ConvergenceWarning:
          lbfgs failed to converge (status=1):
          STOP: TOTAL NO. of ITERATIONS REACHED LIMIT.

          Increase the number of iterations (max_iter) or scale the data as shown in:
              https://scikit-learn.org/stable/modules/preprocessing.html
          Please also refer to the documentation for alternative solver options:
              https://scikit-learn.org/stable/modules/linear_model.html#logistic-regression
            n_iter_i = _check_optimize_result(

Out[89]:  LogisticRegression()

In [90]:  train_predict = logreg.predict(train_x)
          train_predict[:50]

Out[90]:  array(['Arhar/Tur', 'Bajra', 'Sunflower', 'Sunflower', 'Sunflower',
                 'Sunflower', 'Ragi', 'Arhar/Tur', 'Sunflower', 'Ragi', 'Groundnut',
                 'Sunflower', 'Banana', 'Onion', 'Sugarcane', 'Arhar/Tur',
                 'Sunflower', 'Sunflower', 'Groundnut', 'Arhar/Tur', 'Arhar/Tur',
                 'Sunflower', 'Sunflower', 'Arhar/Tur', 'Arhar/Tur', 'Sunflower',
                 'Ragi', 'Rice', 'Sugarcane', 'Arhar/Tur', 'Sunflower', 'Sunflower',
                 'Groundnut', 'Rice', 'Ragi', 'Banana', 'Sunflower', 'Rice',
                 'Arhar/Tur', 'Sunflower', 'Arhar/Tur', 'Sugarcane', 'Arhar/Tur',
                 'Sunflower', 'Groundnut', 'Arhar/Tur', 'Sunflower', 'Sunflower',
                 'Bajra', 'Ragi'], dtype=object)

In [91]:  pd.DataFrame(data1['Crop']).head()
```

FIGURE 6.22   Output of logistic regression algorithm.

6.9   CONCLUSION

This chapter represents a crop selection technique named ECSM (enhanced crop selection model). This method is helpful in the selection of the crop in a particular region and in a particular climatic condition. ECSM takes the weather type, region, state, district, soil type and water density, as these are the important factors that affect crop production. So our proposed model resolves the problem of crop selection by considering all required parameters like soil type, climatic conditions, state, district and water content of the soil. By this, our model can predict the proper crop which is best suited for that particular field and increase the crop production in that given area.

REFERENCES

1. D. E. Rumelhart, G. E. Hinton, and R. J. Williams, "Learning internal representation by error propagation," vol. 1, chapter 8, pp. 418–362. The MIT Press, Cambridge, MA, 1986.

2. J. R. Quinlan, "Learning with continuous classes," in *Proceedings of AI92, 5th Australian Joint Conference on Artificial Intelligence* (Adams & Sterling, eds), pp. 343–348. World Scientific, Singapore, 1992.

3. L. Breiman, J. H. Friedman, R. A. Olshen, and C. J. Stone, *Classification and Regression Trees*. Wadsworth, Belmont, CA, 1984.

4. S. Iniyan, R. Jebakumar, P. Mangalraj, M. Mayank, and N. Aroop, "Plant disease identification and detection using support vector machines and artificial neural networks," in S. S. Dash, C. Lakshmi, S. Das, and B. K. Panigrahi (eds), *Artificial Intelligence and Evolutionary Computations in Engineering Systems AISC 2020* (Vol. 1056), pp. 15–27. Springer, 2020.

5. Rakesh Kumar, M. P. Singh, Prabhat Kumar, and J. P. Singh, "Crop selection method to maximize crop yield rate using machine learning technique," in *2015 International Conference on Smart Technologies and Management for Computing, Communication, Controls, Energy and Materials (ICSTM)*, pp. 138–145, 6–8 May 2015.

6. Karandeep Kaur, "Machine learning: Applications in Indian agriculture," *International Journal of Advanced Research in Computer and Communication Engineering*, Vol. 5, no. 4, April 2016.

7. S. M. Paras, A. Kumar, and M. Chandra, "A feature based neural network model for weather forecasting," *International Journal of Computational Intelligence*, Vol. 4, no. 3, pp. 209–216, 2009.

8. K. Kumar, K. Rupa Kumar, R. G. Ashrit, N. R. Deshpande, and J. W. Hansen, "Climate impacts on Indian agriculture," *International Journal of Climatology*, Vol. 24, p. 13751393, 2004.

9. A. A. Raorane, and R. V. Kulkarni, "Data mining: An effective tool for yield estimation in the agricultural sector," *International Journal of Emerging Trends & Technology in Computer Science (IJETTCS)*, Vol. 1, no. 2, 2012.

10. H. Navarro-Hell, J. Martinez-del Rincon, R. Domingo-Miguel, F. SotoValles, and R. Torres-Sanchez, "A decision support system for managing irrigation in agriculture," *Computers and Electronics in Agriculture*, Vol. 124, pp. 121–131, 2016.

11. E. Khosla, R. Dharavath, and R. Priya, "Crop yield prediction using aggregated rainfall-based modular artificial neural networks and support vector regression," *Environment, Development and Sustainability*, pp. 1–22, 2019.

12. R. Priya, D. Ramesh, and E. Khosla, "Crop prediction on the region belts of India: A naive bayes map reduce precision agricultural model," in *2018 International Conference on Advances in Computing, Communications and Informatics (ICACCI)*, pp. 99–104. IEEE, 2018.

13. R. Kumar, M. Singh, P. Kumar, and J. Singh, "Crop selection method to maximize crop yield rate using machine learning technique," in *2015 International Conference on Smart Technologies and Management for Computing, Communication, Controls, Energy and Materials (ICSTM)*, pp. 138–145. IEEE, 2015.

7 Natural Language Processing Utilisation in Healthcare

S. Vani, Palvadi Srinivas Kumar,
R. Srivel and T. Tangarasan

CONTENTS

7.1 INTRODUCTION

Much advancement is rolling out day by day in the medical domain. At present, we observe that all the super-speciality hospitals and other reputable hospitals are making their patients' records digitised. The healthcare domain is building a wide range in terms of sensors to detect blood pressure, heart rate, oxygen levels in blood, etc. The process of data processing is done by various analyses like lexical analysis, syntax analysis, semantic analysis, intermediate code generator, code optimisation and code generation. Here for processing the patients' information, first, we have to collect the raw data; it may either be structured data or unstructured data (Figure 7.1).

This data is going to be processed and stored in records in a digitised manner; there are many advantages to this, such as security, no paperwork and the ability to track particular patient information by primary key attributes like patient ID. It is

DOI: 10.1201/9781003132110-7

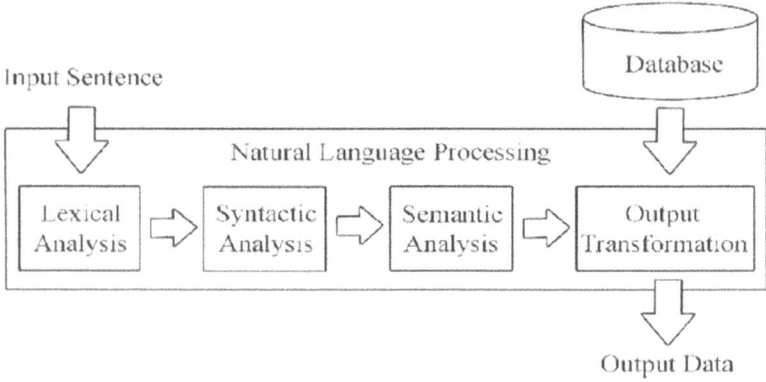

FIGURE 7.1   NLP process.

possible to diagnose the patients' disease based on the symptoms or based on their past health track records. These diagnosis reports help doctors give the proper medication or treatment. Mainly the diagnosis is based on various factors such as patient health record and patient age. By using EHR and NLP techniques we can ensure the best results. Whatever the raw, unstructured or structured data stored in the database for future processing, it should proceed with the following steps: extract, remove negation and code (Figure 7.2).

7.1.1   NATURAL LANGUAGE PROCESSING

We refer to the word NLP, which is used for processing things as a normal person does. By using the NLP mechanism in smart devices, it will perform the task based on the user; examples are Siri and Alexa. Here Siri uses the NLP technique to search the data in the database. By using the NLP mechanism the tasks do not get burdensome; the tasks get digitised which makes the user more comfortable in doing the task.

Natural language processing (NLP) [1] is a mechanism where the data is utilised with the various mechanisms for designing various semantics, computational

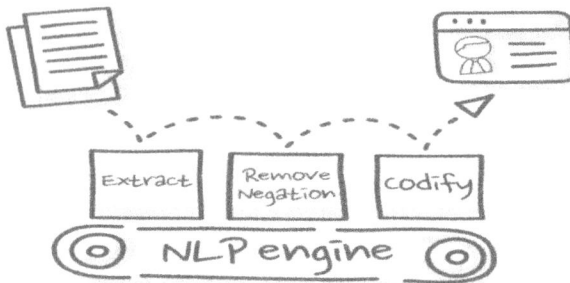

FIGURE 7.2   Data processing procedure.

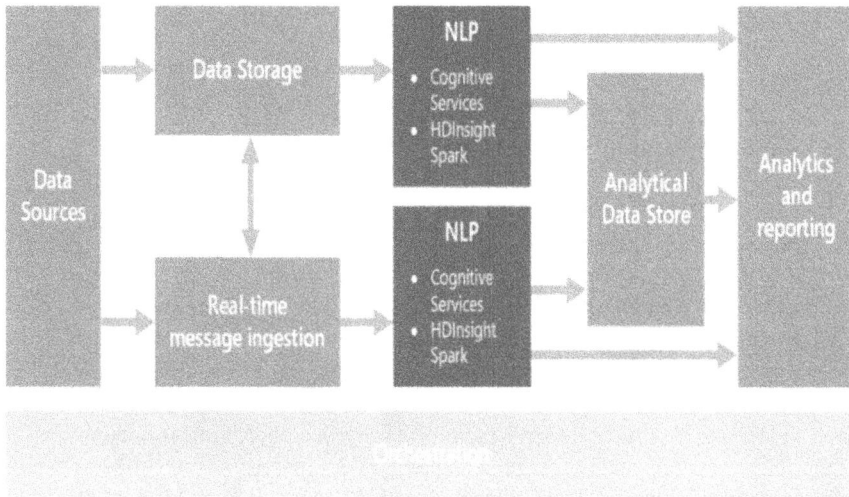

FIGURE 7.3 NLP.

techniques and AI concepts. A lot of data can be done for identifying the things like data collection, data extraction, keyword search and data management. More amounts of the phases and values help identify the phases of the entered data or text (Figure 7.3).

The architecture of NLP has the following characteristics, namely:

- Summarising the given input as either structured data or unstructured data.
- Mapping the raw input as either structured or unstructured data with the patient's record.
- Making the arrangements based on the raw input.
- Making an alert or answer for all types of questions as per our input.

This is the general procedure for the working of NLP as per our request. We have to provide as much raw data or input as possible for better and accurate results. There are several reasons to implement healthcare with NLP, such as identifying the variations among people as well as machines, providing a breakdown, giving the required knowledge, etc.; apart from this, NLP provides many services such as handling the surge in clinical data, supporting vector-based care and health monitoring, improving efficiency, making progress more efficiently, improving patient-to-provider interaction properly, empowering properties, addressing the properties and identifying the patients who need more care. There are further architectures for determining the frameworks of the architecture of NLP, such as:

- Handling a surge in clinical data.
- Supposed value-based care and people's health maintenance.
- Improving clinical documents.

- Making CAC more flexible.
- Improving patients' interaction with EHR.
- Empowering patients with health literacy.
- Addressing the need for high-quality healthcare
- Identifying the patients who need more healthcare.

With NLP the other important thing is EHR. The task of EHR is to make the complete data in digitised form and to make it available to the user whenever needed. Doctors don't generally manage everything well. The extra information input duties make it difficult and can be disappointing. Some doctors experience the ill effects of EHR burnout and take steps to resign from administration early instead of enduring the numerous snaps and screens needed to explore their EHR. Clinical NLP consistently ends up being an answer for this challenge since NLP medical care instruments can undoubtedly get to and precisely decipher clinical documentation. When the erosion of medical care innovation is decreased, we can start to see the value in a greater amount of the advantages of the innovation and less of the everyday dissatisfactions.

The precision of clinical normal language preparing goes up alongside the volume of information accessible for learning. The more a clinical NLP stage is utilised, the more exact utilising computerised reasoning in medical services gets, since it's continually learning and sometimes can be adjustable. Some NLP medical care frameworks offered by sellers promote the capacity to screen how the clinical normal language handling would at first perform with a particular clinical gathering, and then, at that point alter it closer to the requirements of that specific clinical gathering.

A particular benefit that regular language handling clinical records offers is the capacity for PC-helped coding to orchestrate the substance of long outline notes into simply the significant focuses. Verifiably, this could take associations weeks, months or even years to physically audit and interact piles of diagram notes from wellbeing records, just to recognise the appropriate information. Regular language preparation to programme for medical services can check the clinical content in practically no time and distinguish what should be extricated. This opens up doctors and staff assets to zero in on complex matters and decreases the time spent on excess regulatory strategy. At the point when PCs can comprehend doctor documentation precisely and measure that information, likewise, significant choice help can be acquired. These bits of knowledge can be of huge use for future medication research and customised medication, which is useful for patients and suppliers.

Doctors don't all "talk a similar way", and ought to consistently know that their notes and reports will probably be perused by their work friends, patients, and even PCs, as indicated by their association's security strategy. Staying away from non-standard language in note creation and the board is critical [2]. Most normal language-preparing medical care equipment is designed to oblige a wide variety of clinical documentation phrasing. Nonetheless, utilising extraordinary abbreviations can befuddle NLP coding calculations and other clinical note perusers.

In 2018 and 2019 the advancement to improve regular language-handling medical care information has demonstrated testing. On the off chance that the NLP yields show too many proposed ends or fake ends that are erroneous, clients will figure out how to overlook the knowledge and end up with a framework that can diminish in general business efficiency. NLP programming for medical care should revolve around information ends that have the least clamour and the most grounded signal about what medical care suppliers need to do.

Medical care regular language handling offers the opportunity for PCs to do the things that PCs need to do: the examination, the HCC hazard change coding, the administrative centre capacities and the patient set investigation, all without hindering doctor correspondence [3].

NLP in medical care is setting out new and energising open doors for medical services conveyance and patient experience. Soon specific NLP coding acknowledgement empowers doctors to invest more energy with patients while helping make adroit ends dependent on exact information. In the years to come, we'll hear the news, and see the conceivable outcomes of this innovation, as it engages suppliers to decidedly impact wellbeing results. The saddest part of the research is we identified that more than 80% of the data is unstructured and as a result, it is giving poor quality of results. At present, whatever data is collected from the patients is mostly unstructured data. The present major challenging task or goal or agenda is to put unstructured data into a structured order; to do this, we will have to know various characteristics or properties of the text file or image file such as the name of the file, which person the file belongs to, the type of disease mentioned in the file, the medicine given for that patient, patient age, etc., based on the available data in the unstructured database. By applying a few characteristics we can make data in a structured manner [4].

Based on the webinar given by Chendy in 2018, compared to all other types of data, text data is the only challenging task for storing the data in the database. Because the text data occupies more space compared to other documents, the time taken to search entire keywords in text data will be more. Whenever the NLP does the three phases automatically, it starts with classification, extraction and summarisation.

In 2015, the user made a study regarding suicide cases using the NLP technique [5]. They have focused on social media regarding suicide cases. They have identified that many have posted a sad emoji in the form of text and some have posted a blue- or red-coloured broken heart emoji while attempting suicide and very few have posted a red-coloured angry emoji saying that they were angry before suicide [6]. The generated results show 70% accuracy. Based on this survey over Twitter, the author proves that NLP helps in predictive analysis. The other thing NLP can perform is boosting phenotyping capacity, which enables quality improvement.

Apart from many of the advantages, there are a few limitations in NLP; extracting the data from the server from EHR will be easy, but training the dataset is a complex task. Making or understanding the proper meaning from some text is very complicated and takes a lot of time, so the input given to the NLP should be given in proper English language [7] because it can read only English. Incorrect words, incorrect spellings and inappropriate words will not be considered.

7.2 BACKGROUND WORK RELATED TO THIS DOMAIN

Natural language processing is the automatic process in which things will be performed based on suggestions and queries. The help of NLP is going to give the best results for the data which we have searched from the database. The process of natural language processing includes understanding, generation and querying [8].

There are many use-case mechanisms for text classifications at present as well as in future, such as:

- Speech recognition
- Improving patient's data for more accuracy
- Research in stored data
- Various querying techniques in the database for proper results
- Automatic response based on user input
- Ambient virtual scribe
- Biometric discovery
- Population health management and monitoring
- Tech labs
- Speech recognition
- Improving clinical documentation
- Computer-assisted coding
- Automated reporting
- Clinical trials
- Priority authorisation
- Clinical decision support
- Risk adjustment
- Biomarker identification
- People surveillance

Out of all the various kinds of applications, the NLP mechanism gives better and good results in all aspects and has significantly improved healthcare. The development of healthcare using natural language processing is having a good impact, such as in:

- Clinical trial matching
- Prior authorisation
- Decision support for medical data
- Identifying risk and adjusting risks based on that risk criteria

These are the general advancements in the NLP techniques shown in Figure 7.4 [9]. The development in the NLP mechanism is happening in the following terms:

- Improving the patient's health record by directly interacting with patients
- Increasing awareness of patients
- Improving the quality of health records
- Improving care quality
- Identifying the care and identifying the critical needs

7.2.1 ARCHITECTURE OF NATURAL LANGUAGE PROCESSING UTILISATION IN HEALTHCARE

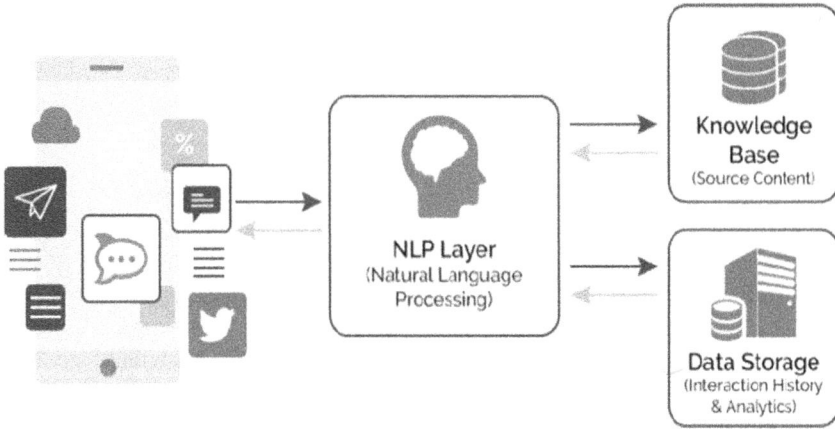

FIGURE 7.4 NLP in healthcare.

7.2.2 IMPLEMENTATION AND RESULTS OF HEALTHCARE USING NLP

To perform the NLP technique in the healthcare domain, we have to collect the history of the patient's health record as much as possible [10]. Here, the more information is available for the patient, the more accurate results we can generate for the diagnosis of the patient. The following is the procedure for how the data is processed.

Step 1: Enter the patient records in devices.
Step 2: Save the data in the server in the proper entity order.
Step 3: Decision support system.
Step 4: From the above-entered data, search in terms of values or entities or names or disease or age.
Steps 5: Now based on the patient's health problems, assess the situation and the medication.
Step 6: Assess various factors such as quality, risk for the patient and efficiency in the generated results as well as safety for the patient which were stored in the server.
Step 7: Assess value, impact, benefit, impact or quality, efficiency, risk and safety.
Step 8: Perform Step 4 and Step 7 repeatedly.

We have designed this mechanism only in the English language and we have made this information by taking hybrid datasets of patients. The controlling mechanism was performed on the data which is present in the datasets.

The data processing will be performed in the following phases: data extraction and data analysis.

7.2.3   DATA EXTRACTION

Data extraction will be done based on the phrases or keywords like first name, last name, surname. Here the risk level (RL), as well as the confidence level (CL), was generated based on the patient's medical history. After the data collection, the CL and difference in the mean values were calculated [11]. These generated values will be considered after taking two reviews and having a discussion with the patient.

7.2.4   DATA ANALYSIS

Whatever results were generated with analysis, for the outcome results, metadata was generated. The outcome results were performed with various values, settings and pairs. Here various results were generated for various patients' records, which we can call heterogeneity data [12]. Here data will be formed into groups as well as subgroups. Here the generated results will be tested with the individual studies to check the efficiency in the results. Based on the results the risk assessment or the change in the predictions is identified (Figure 7.5).

At present more than 60 companies are working in the medical domain for various tasks such as data gathering, data filtration, data security, access permissions, etc. The main agenda for working on the patients' data is to make patients' data into a database [13] so that while searching based on keywords or by search criteria, the results can be generated more efficiently and accurately.

7.2.5   ROLE OF NLP OR DEEP LEARNING IN HEALTHCARE

As per the general terms, the classification is divided into four phases, namely doctor, patient, paramedical staff and pharmaceuticals (Table 7.1).

After this process completes for every image, it will perform the map-reduce operation to see the relevant images or the matching image which [14] already exists in the database. This map-reduce will be performed with any type of data like text, image audio or video (Figure 7.6).

In healthcare, this mechanism is used in making quick and accurate decisions and also gives the best summary to the patient based upon the health problems of the patient. This mechanism helps in making clinical decisions for medication purposes or for diagnosis purposes. The NLP mechanism needs the support of EHR for making the process run in a smooth manner. The outstanding research done in 2019 defines that when the doctor treated 100 patients at the same time, the NLP with the support of the EHR technique gave medication to 1,000 people based upon their disease with 96.13% accuracy.

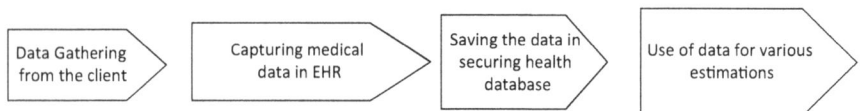

Data Gathering from the client → Capturing medical data in EHR → Saving the data in securing health database → Use of data for various estimations

FIGURE 7.5   Electronic health record evolution for data analysis.

TABLE 7.1

Healthcare Data Stages

Sr. No.	Situation	Process	Tools/Devices/Reports/Actions
1	Pre-disease	Health awareness	Smart sensor devices to provide health updates
		Regular health check-ups	Devices for health check-ups
		How to stay away from disease?	Training programmes and devices for various exercises
2	In-disease	Diagnosis	Blood sample, X-ray image, urine sample, biopsy, devices for checking vital signs in the body (oxygen, sugar, heartbeat, pulse, etc.)
		Treatment	Pre-surgery treatments, minor surgery, major surgery, combined surgery, post-surgery treatments
		Medication	Drug dosage based on the nature of the body for a single disease, multiple diseases
3	Post-disease	Follow-ups	Prediction of the number of follow-ups or time period of follow-ups required
		Improvement comparison	Compare pre-, in- and post-disease reports
		Future predictions	

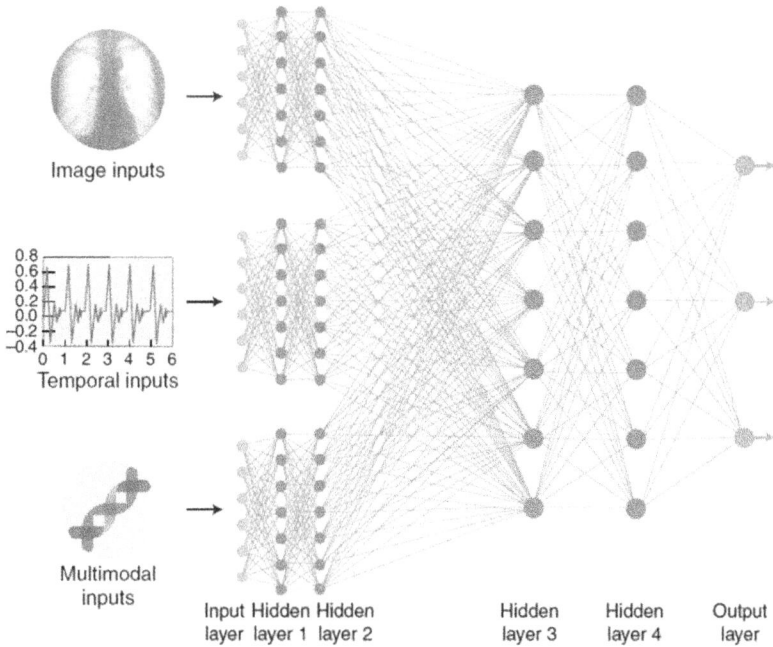

FIGURE 7.6 Map-reduce procedure.

7.2.6   How Healthcare Organisations Use NLP at Present

We have to start the task in NLP with low-level problems and then higher-level problems. Whatever requests are coming for processing, we have to process the task and deliver the result based on search criteria. When NLP is processing for one task, like for a headache, it should only give the result to the searched keyword. The study defined that compared to unstructured data the structured data gives more accurate data [15]. The following are the things we have to follow while designing the NLP, like interphases, ambitious vocabulary and semantic roles.

7.2.6.1   Interphases

In the event that a clinician needs to know whether a patient has social help yet the expression "has social help" isn't in the EHR, cutting-edge NLP will actually want to gather importance from the unique circumstance [16]. Rather than depending on the specific expression of "has social help", the framework will deal with an expression like "sibling at the bedside" and realise it implies the patient has social help.

7.2.6.2   Ambitious Vocabulary

In the event that an examiner programmes the NLP framework to search for the expression "sibling at the bedside" and it sees the expression "remained at the bedside" or "sibling kicked the bucket of cardiovascular failure", it will realise that the significance isn't something similar in spite of one of the words being in something similar. With current NLP frameworks, these two expressions would bring back bogus positives for importance equivalent to "sibling at the bedside".

7.2.6.3   Semantic Roles

The current NLP framework battles with semantic jobs. The expression "spouse assists patient with medications" is altogether different from "patient assists wife with prescriptions". However, a watchword-based NLP [17] framework can't separate between the two expressions, which is a current constraint of NLP. Later, NLP frameworks could be customised to comprehend semantic jobs (e.g. what's the subject and who's the article) (Figure 7.7).

NLP is getting more advancement in brain-related problems. Using the NLP technique helps in detecting the brain clots of a person. They have been identified with the help of more than 25 brain-imaging pictures [18] which has given positive values for cerebrovascular and neuron-degenerative phenotypes. The NLP technique works based on the XML-based training of the text data (Figure 7.8).

7.3   CONCLUSION

Deep learning in NLP is playing a major role in making decisions for the users or patients based on the search criteria. NLP is promising to gather even more data than what it has in order to improve the quality of the given input or the best suggestion technique based on the given input. Many of the techniques came into existence by integrating with the current existing trends for better performance. We have done a

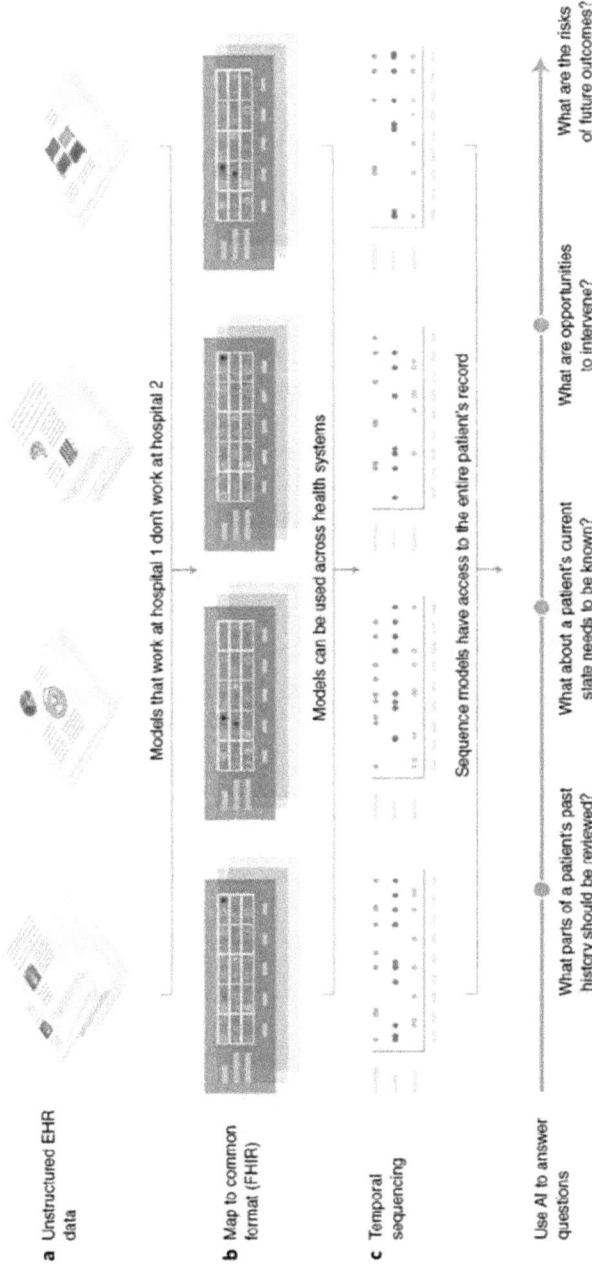

FIGURE 7.7   Making predictions using EHR.

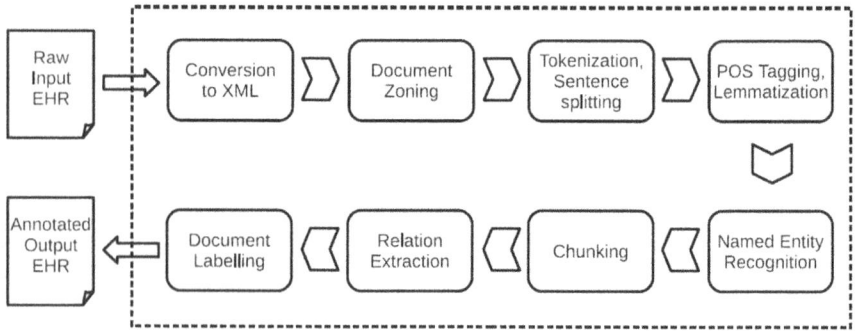

FIGURE 7.8 EDIE architecture.

lot of analysis of the NLP mechanism in the domain of healthcare. For designing this chapter we have taken various terms and conditions for the development of the work. The NLP technique helps to improve the lot in the clinical data for making better decisions and critical decisions in time and helps doctors make quick decisions. Several mechanisms were improved in the NLP in the domain of healthcare for better and more accurate results. Overall by studying the concept of healthcare using NLP we observed two major difficulties, namely data access and data assessment; calculating the detailed data and making access permissions with prior security is a challenging task. The NLP technique for the assessment of patients is improving the quality of service and exactness in the data.

REFERENCES

1. Yang, J.-J.; Li, J.; Mulder, J.; Wang, Y.; Chen, S.; Wu, H.; Wang, Q.; Pan, H. Emerging information technologies for enhanced healthcare. *Comput. Ind.* 2015, 69, 3–11.
2. Cortada, J.W.; Gordon, D.; Lenihan, B. *The Value of Analytics in Healthcare*; Report No.: GBE03476-USEN-00; IBM Institute for Business Value, Armonk, NY, 2012.
3. Prokosch, H.-U.; Ganslandt, T. Perspectives for medical informatics. *Methods Inf. Med.* 2009, 48, 38–44.
4. Simpao, A.F.; Ahumada, L.M.; Gálvez, J.A.; Rehman, M.A. A review of analytics and clinical informatics in health care. *J. Med. Syst.* 2014, 38, 45.
5. Ghassemi, M.; Celi, L.A.; Stone, D.J. State of the art review: The data revolution in critical care. *Crit. Care* 2015, 19, 118.
6. Tomar, D.; Agarwal, S. A survey on data mining approaches for healthcare. *Int. J. Bio-Sci. Bio-Technol.* 2013, 5, 241–266.
7. Huang, Y.; McCullagh, P.; Black, N.; Harper, R. Feature selection and classification model construction on type 2 diabetic patients' data. *Artif. Intell. Med.* 2007, 41, 251–262.
8. Althoff, T.; Clark, K.; Leskovec, J. Natural language processing for mental health: Large scale discourse analysis of counseling conversations, *CoRR*. abs/1605.04462.
9. Sparck Jones, K. Evaluating natural language processing systems: An analysis and review, lecture notes in computer science. *Lect. Notes Arti. Intel.* 1995, 1083.
10. Paroubek, P.; Chaudiron, S.; Hirschman, L. Editorial: Principles of evaluation in natural language processing. *TAL*, 2007, 48(1), 7–31. http://www.atala.org/Editorial.

11. Dybkjaer, L. *Evaluation of Text and Speech Systems, Text, Speech and Language Technology*, 2007, 37.
12. Wu, S.; Miller T.; Masanz, J.; Coarr, M.; Halgrim, S.; Carrell, D.; Clark, C. Negation's notsolved: Generalizability versus optimizability in clinical natural language processing. *PLOS One* 2014, 9(11), 1–11. https://doi.org/10.1371/journal.pone.0112774.
13. Demner-Fushman, D.; Chapman, W.W.; McDonald, C.J. What can natural language processing do for clinical decision support? *J. Biomed. Inform.* 2009, 42(5), 760–772.
14. Zheng, K.; Vydiswaran, V.G.V.; Liu, Y.; Wang, Y.; Stubbs, A.; Uzuner, O.; Gururaj, A.E.; Bayer, S.; Aberdeen, J.; Rumshisky, A.; Pakhomov, S.; Liu, H.; Xu, H. Ease of adoptionof clinical natural language processing software: An evaluation of five systems. *J. Biomed. Inform.* 2015, 58 Suppl, S189–96.
15. Kaufman, D.R.; Sheehan, B.; Stetson, P.; Bhatt, A.R.; Field, A.I.; Patel, C.; Maisel, J.M. Natural language processing-enabled and conventional data capture methods forinput to electronic health records: A comparative usability study. *JMIR Med. Inform.* 2016, 4 (4), e35.
16. Suominen, H.; Zhou, L.; Hanlen, L.; Ferraro, G. Benchmarking clinical speech recognitionand information extraction: New data, methods, and evaluations. *JMIR Med. Inform.* 2015, 3(2), e19.
17. Aramaki, E.; Morita, M.; Kano, Y.; Ohkuma, T. Overview of the NTCIR-11 MedNLPtask. In *Proceedings of the 11th NTCIR Conference, NII Testbeds and Community for Information Access Research (NTCIR)*, Tokyo, Japan, 2014, 147–154.
18. Rangasamy, S.; Nadenichek, R.; Rayasam, M.; Sozdatelev, A. *Natural Language Processing in Healthcare*. December 6, 2018.

8 Traffic Management in 5G Networks
Case Studies

*G. Kavitha, P. Rupa Ezhil Arasi, G. Kalaimani
and Palvadi Srinivas Kumar*

CONTENTS

8.1 5G NETWORKS

5G is a new global wireless standard for mobile networks. 5G network connects machines, objects and devices virtually together. The major advantages of 5G networks are high reliability, more network capacity, increased availability, low latency, higher performance, improved efficiency, etc. 5G networks also provide users with new experiences and the networks establish connections with new industries.

The first-generation (1G) mobile network supported analogue devices for communication. Communication through digital voice was bought into existence in the second-generation (2G) network through the usage of code-division multiple access (CDMA) technology. Mobile data was introduced in the third generation (3G), and the fourth-generation (4G) mobile network paved the way for mobile broadband service. 5G technology provides more connectivity than the existing mobile networks.

DOI: 10.1201/9781003132110-8

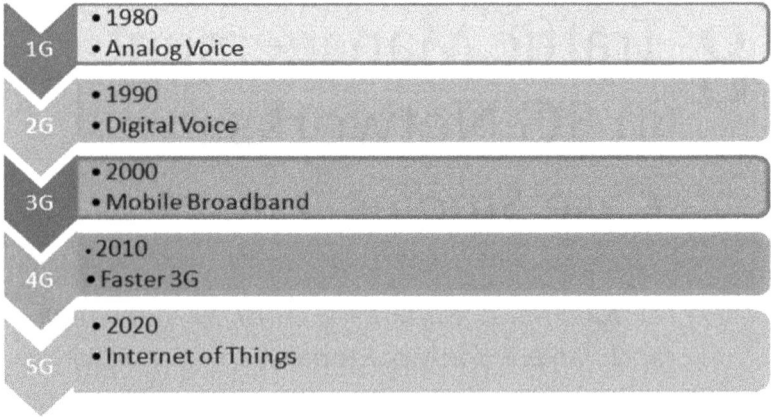

FIGURE 8.1 Evolution of 5G.

The technologies such as mobile broadband, mission-critical services and the Internet of Things contributed to the evolution of 5G technology (Figure 8.1).

8.1.1 5G NETWORK ARCHITECTURE

The 5G network employs radio access networks (RAN) in its architecture [1]. Hence, 5G network is not complex and has an intelligent infrastructure. The intelligent network is updated with functional architecture, new host interfaces and protocols. The main transformations in the 5G network are radio access networks, new core and operations with massive MIMO antenna systems. The frequency range will be from 450 MHz to approximately 50 GHz (Figure 8.2).

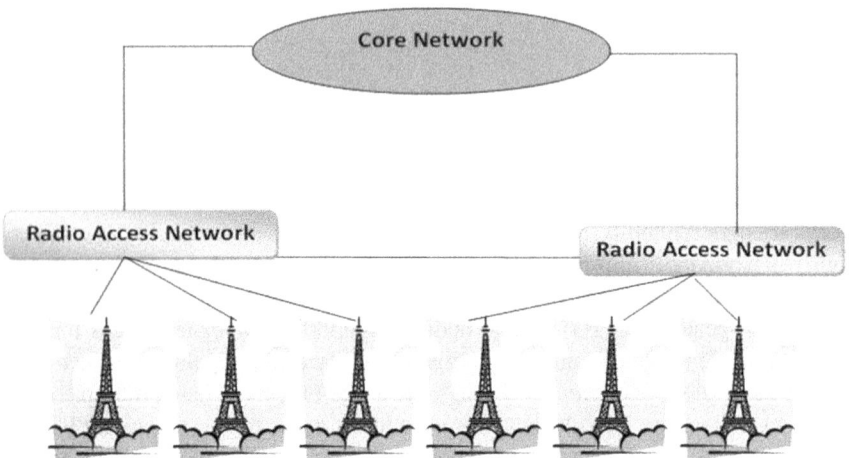

FIGURE 8.2 5G network architecture.

The radio access network (*RAN*) is formed by connecting various cells, mobile towers, systems, etc. The RAN then establishes the connection with the core network. The main responsibility of the *core network* is to supervise the connections that exist among data, voice, etc. The core network provides faster response time by integrating itself with various cloud-based services. The functionalities of the core network include network virtualisation, network application slicing and so on.

8.1.2   NEED FOR 5G NETWORK

The world today is a cellular world and there is always a need for data management, network management and so on. Industries and organisations are in need of the fastest network and this led to the evolution of 5G. 5G extends the reach of mobile broadband and hence it supports virtual reality, autonomous vehicle technology and also provides improved data and network security.

8.1.3   BENEFITS OF 5G NETWORK

a. The Internet of Things connects billions of devices and 5G paves way for machine-to-machine communication in the interconnected network. This advancement laid the foundations for revolutions in various fields such as agriculture, education, healthcare, etc.
b. 5G provides ultra-reliable low-latency communications. This is advantageous for remote medical care, treatments, robotics and automation and various safety systems.
c. 5G networks provide more increased broadband than any other network. Hence the data are transferred at a faster rate.
d. The 5G network enables downloading and streaming content with high speed hence it provides faster speeds in data access.
e. 5G provides spontaneous interconnections between the devices and hence offers enhanced computing power.
f. With new 5G technology, the mobile spectrum is increased and shows a radio frequency range above 6 GHz.
g. The 5G network has greater capacity and covers a wide range of devices.

8.1.4   5G APPLICATIONS

The 5G network plays a vital role in various applications such as healthcare, transport, industrial automation, virtual and augmented reality, etc. (Figure 8.3).

8.1.5   5G REQUIREMENTS

5G network architecture transfers data at a 10 Gbps data rate in one-millisecond latency. The network covers a higher number of devices and provides a battery life of more than ten years (Figure 8.4).

5G

Transport

Health Care

Industrial Automation

Virtual and Augmented
Reality

Smart City

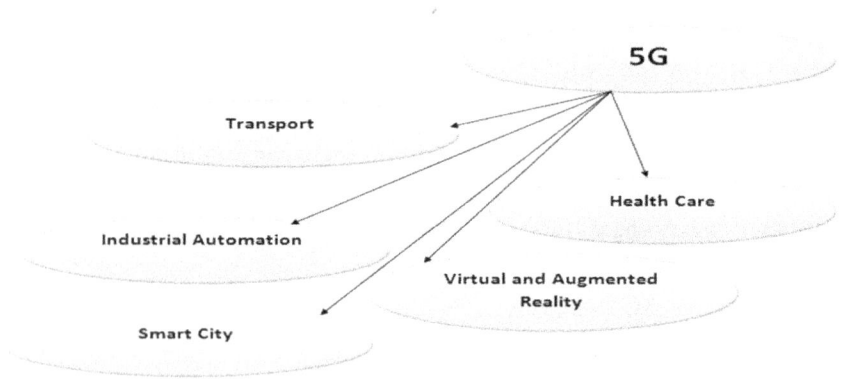

FIGURE 8.3 Applications of 5G.

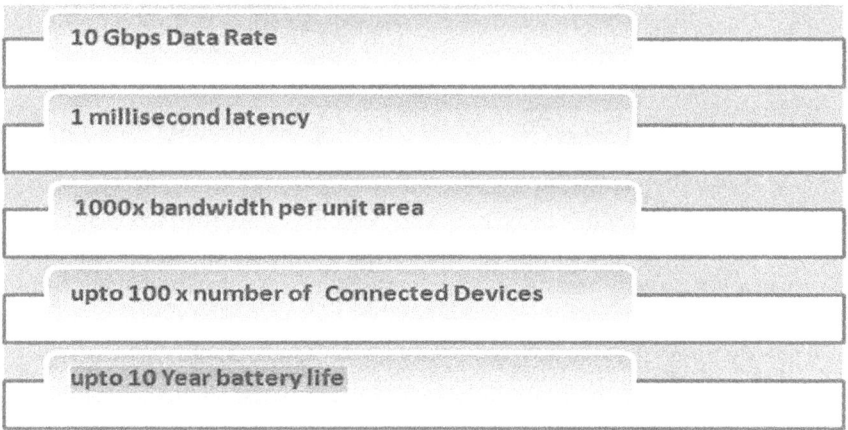

10 Gbps Data Rate

1 millisecond latency

1000x bandwidth per unit area

upto 100 x number of Connected Devices

upto 10 Year battery life

FIGURE 8.4 Requirements of 5G.

8.2   ARTIFICIAL INTELLIGENCE AND 5G NETWORKS

Artificial intelligence (AI) enables machines to think and act like human beings. In recent times 5G and AI have been the most innovative technologies. Employing AI to improve the performance of mobile networks also solves the existing issues in wireless technology which cannot be solved using traditional methods.

AI has a strong effect on 5G network management. AI improves the quality of service, simplifies deployment, provides higher network efficiency and improves network security [2]. AI also detects various issues in the network infrastructure (Figure 8.5).

The objective of 5G networks is to provide a low-latency, high-speed network that connects a massive number of devices. AI and machine learning (ML) complement 5G networks with autonomous operations that transform 5G into a scalable real-time network. AI and ML can be used in all the layers of the 5G network, from the radio

Mobility Management   Self Organizing Networks

User Behavior Prediction   Improved Network
                                                            Security

                              5 G

Congestion Control and Routing

                                          User Localization

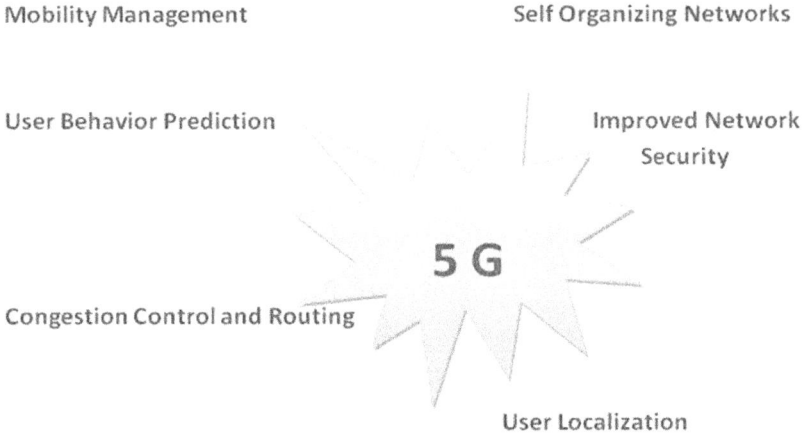

FIGURE 8.5   AI and 5G technology.

access layer to the integrated access backhaul (IAB) and then to the distributed cloud
(core) layer. Hence, AI and ML complement 5G technology in network planning,
automating network operations, network slicing, reducing operating costs, etc.

8.2.1   AI in the Radio Access Network Layer

AI and ML, when implemented in RAN, improve the network's performance in
three domains: network design, network optimisation and RAN algorithms. The
RAN performance optimisation depends upon the parameters utilised, the type
and number of network objects involved and the frequency at which the network
is updated. The performance optimisation is obtained when RAN algorithms are
replaced by AI controllers (Figure 8.6).

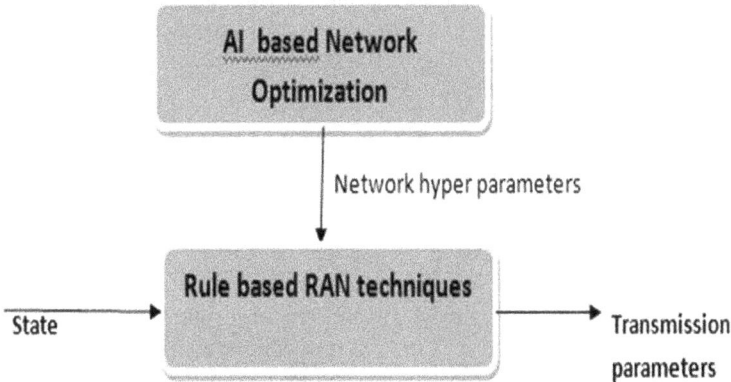

AI based Network
Optimization

Network hyper parameters

State   Rule based RAN techniques

                                                  Transmission
                                                  parameters

FIGURE 8.6   AI for RAN optimisation.

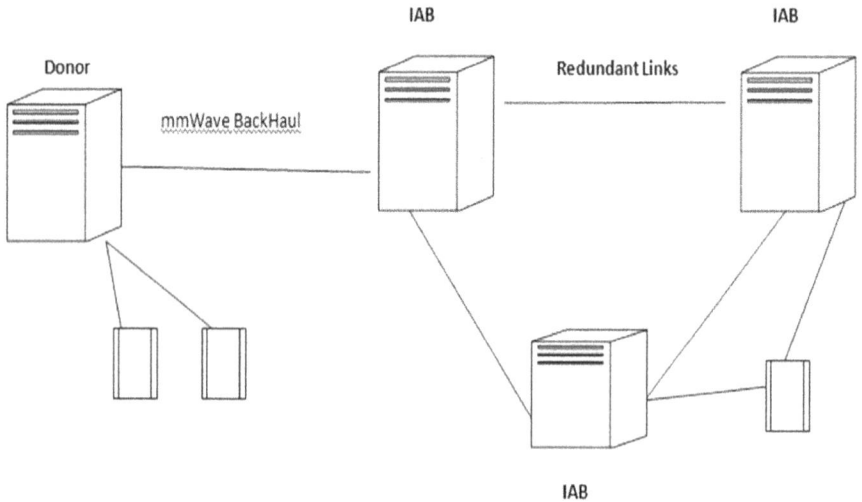

FIGURE 8.7   Integrated access backhaul (IAB).

8.2.2   AI IN THE INTEGRATED ACCESS BACKHAUL (IAB) LAYER

The objective of the IAB network layer is to provide 5G networks at millimetre Wave frequencies (mmWave) and AI can be utilised for improving the performance of the IAB network layer (Figure 8.7).

8.2.3   AI IN THE CORE LAYER

In the core layer, AI and ML can be utilised for system resource optimisation, auto-scaling, anamoly detection, predictive analysis, prescriptive policies, etc.

In general, AI and ML, when integrated with 5G networks, help in network resource management, network security optimisation, traffic management, fault prediction and system monitoring. Machine learning algorithms consist of representation, evaluation and optimisation techniques to enhance the performance of 5G networks.

8.3   DEEP LEARNING IN 5G NETWORKS

Deep learning (DL) is a subset of machine learning techniques that extracts features automatically from the given dataset. The extracted features are utilised by a DNN (deep neural network) in classifying the mobile data and in decision-making. In 5G networks, DL is utilised for predicting and classifying the mobile applications, generating network slices, making routing decisions, providing network security and so on.

A convolution neural network (CNN) is a special type of deep neural network (DNN) capable of handling large volumes of data [3]. CNN is based upon mathematical models such as convolutions and linear operations. CNN is mainly utilised for traffic flow prediction in 5G networks and object classification.

A recurrent neural network (RNN) [3] uses long short-term memory to recollect the information learned in the previous steps in addition to the inputs. RNN provides a solution for mobility issues and helps in traffic prediction in 5G networks.

8.3.1 RESEARCH CHALLENGES

Deep learning is utilised to detect the issues in a 5G network at various levels. At the physical level, DL addresses channel state information (CSI) estimation, fault detection, device location prediction, coding/decoding scheme representation, radiofrequency characterisation, multi-user detection, self-interference and radio parameter definition and beamforming definition. DL at the network level can be utilised for traffic prediction and anomaly detection. Finally, at the application level, DL techniques can be utilised for the characterisation of applications. But there are various issues and challenges in integrating DL with 5G networks (Figure 8.8).

The challenges in integrating DL and 5G networks are [4]:

a. Designing and developing mathematical models using DL is very difficult.
b. DL models are capable of processing a large variety of data but the solutions proposed offer only low computational complexity.

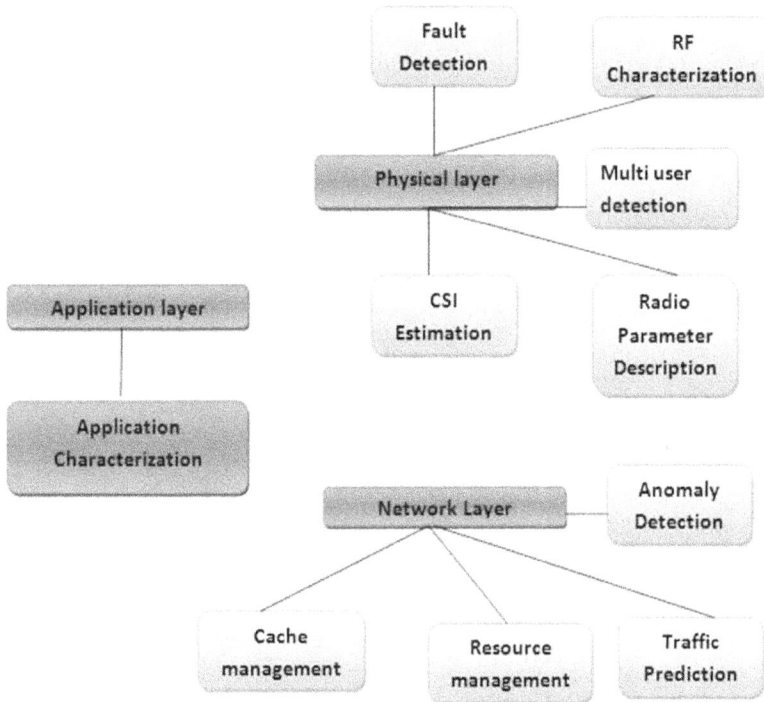

FIGURE 8.8 Research challenges identified in 5G networks.

    c. The inclusion of new parameters might have an effect on network performance.

    d. Deep learning techniques can be utilised only for networks with massive connections and the processing power of the devices might influence the utilisation.

8.3.2 Deep Learning–Based Traffic Prediction in 5G Networks

The evolution of modern communication media and 5G networks has led to the growth of traffic data. Managing Internet traffic is the challenge to be faced by researchers in the near future.

Traditional network traffic prediction methods are ineffective in handling the huge volume of network traffic data [5]. Hence, the solution is to design a network architecture that optimises available network resources by employing appropriate scheduling techniques, thereby minimising energy consumption and avoiding the issues in the underlying network structure.

From the literature, it is evident that a proactive network slice technique integrated with deep learning can be utilised for network traffic prediction [6]. A deep learning model based on spatial and temporal dependencies can also be utilised to predict traffic [7]. Hence, a mobile traffic dataset when investigated using a deep learning neural network [8] can classify the traffic as low, medium or high. CNN and RNN can be merged and utilised to extract geographical and temporal traffic features and predict the type of traffic (Figure 8.9).

The RNN [9] model comprises a regression stage and a feature extraction stage. This RNN model accepts traffic data predicted at the final hour as its inputs. Then, various DL models can be utilised for feature extraction from the inputs. The features thus extracted are passed to the regression layer. The upper layer provides the output values (Figure 8.10).

The 3D-CNN model [10] along with the spatial and temporal information also utilises the time for traffic prediction. The CNN model consists of three pooling

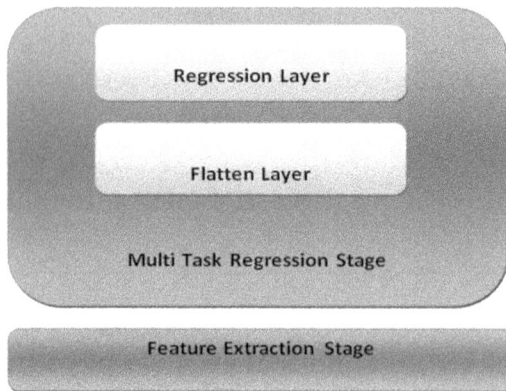

FIGURE 8.9 Recurrent neural network (RNN) model for traffic prediction.

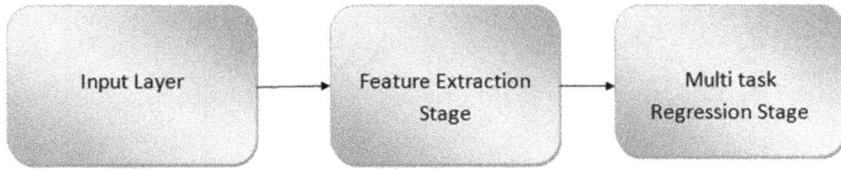

FIGURE 8.10 3D-CNN model for traffic prediction.

layers and three convolution layers. The kernel size parameters and the number of kernels vary in each convolution layer similar to stride size and pooling policy.

The 3D-CNN model [11, 12] suits the spatial domain and the RNN model suits the time domain. The combined RNN and 3D-CNN model description is given in Figure 8.11.

Convolution layers are chosen from among {32, 64, 128, 256, 512, 1,024}. Kernel and strides in convolutional and pooling layers are given as {k,k}, where the value of k is between 1 and 6. The pooling policy is average pooling or max pooling. LSTM cells in RNN are chosen from among {32, 64, 128, 256, 512, 1,024}. The number of layers in RNN is chosen from between 1 and 4 (Figure 8.12).

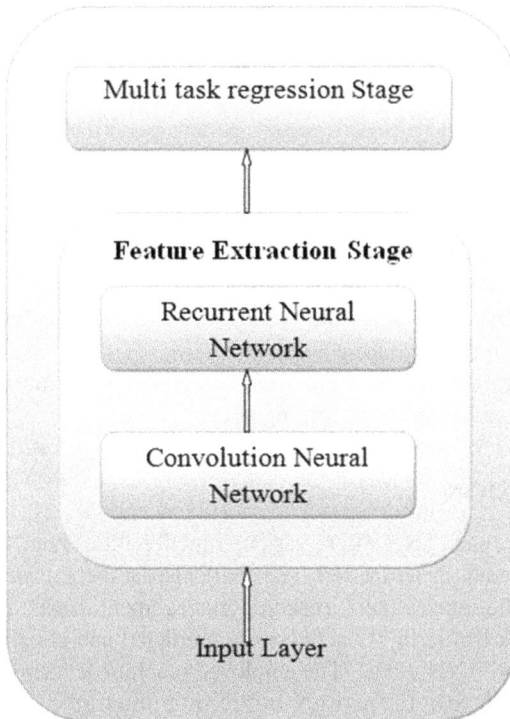

FIGURE 8.11 RNN and 3D-CNN combined model for traffic prediction.

	Layer	Cells	Cell Type	Steps
Recurrent Neural Network	Layer 1	256	LSTM	6
	Layer 2	256	LSTM	6

	Layer	No. of kernels	Kernel Size	Stride size	Pooling Policy
Convolution Neural Network	Convolution 1	64	5,5	1,1	
	Pooling 1		2,2	2,2	Maximum
	Convolution 2	128	5,5	1,1	
	Pooling 2		2,2	2,2	Average
	Convolution 3	64	5,5	1,1	
	Pooling 3		2,2	1,1	Average

FIGURE 8.12   The hyperparameters for RNN and 3D-CNN.

At the multitask regression stage the traffic falls under any of the following three categories:

- Maximum traffic: Refers to the maximum traffic value among the six network traffic values in the upcoming hour.
- Average traffic: Represents the average of network values predicted every ten minutes in the upcoming hour.
- Minimum traffic: Refers to the minimum traffic value among the six network traffic values in the upcoming hour.

8.4   CONCLUSION

In the 5G network, each layer offers various functionalities but there are still some challenges that need to be addressed. The challenges at the network layer are anomaly detection, cache management, resource management, traffic prediction, etc. In this work, network traffic in 5G networks is predicted and classified using a combined 3D-CNN and RNN model. The employed machine learning techniques accurately predict and classify the network traffic from the traffic data stored. Thus by using combined RNN and 3D-CNN for traffic prediction, the traffic loads can be predicted and classified as maximum, minimum or average.

REFERENCES

1. Metin Ozturk, Mandar Gogate, Muhammad A. Imran, Oluwakayode Onireti, Ahsan Adeel, Amir Hussain, "A novel deep learning driven, low-cost mobility prediction approach for 5G cellular networks: The case of the Control/Data Separation Architecture (CDSA)", *Neurocomputing* 358 (2019), pp:479–489.
2. Hao Meng, Wasswa Shafik, S. Mojtaba Matinkhah, Zubair Ahmad, "A 5G beam selection machine learning algorithm for unmanned aerial vehicle applications", *Wireless Communications and Mobile Computing* 2020 (2020), pp:1–16.
3. Miranda McClellan, Cristina Cervelló-Pastor, Sebastià Sallent, "Deep learning at the mobile edge: Opportunities for 5G networks", *Journal of Applied Sciences* 10 (2020), pp:1–27.
4. M. Li, H. Li, "Application of deep neural network and deep reinforcement learning in wireless communication", *PLOS ONE* 15 (2020), pp:1–15.
5. Mahmoud Abbasi, Amin Shahraki, Amir Taherkordi, "Deep learning for network traffic monitoring and analysis (NTMA): A survey", *Computer Communications* 170 (2021), pp:19–41.
6. Alberto Mozo, Bruno Ordozgoiti, Sandra Gómez-Canaval, "Forecasting short-term data center network traffic load with convolutional neural networks", February 6 (2018), https://doi.org/10.1371/journal.pone.0191939.
7. Lan Liu, Jun Lin, Pengcheng Wang, Langzhou Liu, Rongfu Zhou, "Deep learning-based network security data sampling and anomaly prediction in future network", *Discrete Dynamics in Nature and Society* 2020 (2020), p:4163825, https://doi.org/10.1155/2020/4163825.
8. Imad Alawe, Adlen Ksentini, Yassine Hadjadj-Aoul, Philippe Bertin, "Improving traffic forecasting for 5G core network scalability: A machine learning approach", *IEEE Network Magazine*, IEEE (2018), pp:1–10.
9. Chih-Wei Huang, Chiu-Ti Chiang, Qiuhui Li, "A study of deep learning networks on mobile traffic forecasting", *IEEE Conference Proceedings* (2017), pp:1–6.
10. R. Raturi, A. Kumar, "An analytical approach for health data analysis and finding the correlations of attributes using decision tree and W-logistic modal process", *IJIRCCE* 7(6) (2019), ISSN (Online): 2320-9801, ISSN (Print): 23209798.
11. S. Chandrasekaran, A. Kumar, "Implementing medical data processing with Ann with hybrid approach of implementation", *Journal of Advanced Research in Dynamical and Control Systems – JARDCS* 10(10) (2018), pp:45–52.
12. Djamel Sadok Guto Leoni Santos, Patricia Takako Endo, Judith Kelner, "When 5G meets deep learning: A systematic review", *Journal of Algorithms* 13 (2020), pp:1–34.

9 Big Data–Based Frameworks and Machine Learning

Kesana Mohana Lakshmi and
Tummala Ranga Babu

CONTENTS

9.1 INTRODUCTION

Image is an essential part of daily life [1]. As technology is increasing rapidly everything is getting digitalised and the best way to preserve the most valuable ancient manuscripts and literature is to convert printed text into the form of a digital document. Acknowledgement of words from revealed Telugu files is now no longer being investigated a great deal, in contrast with the commonplace files in English. Therefore there is reduction in the efficiency, facts and also the precision. On the opposite hand, characters in south Indian scripts like Telugu are composed of multiple items, making it more complicated to use an excessive degree of characteristic extraction techniques. Therefore, there is a need for alternative methods apart from the existing traditional methods as per the literature. The existing schemes are best suited for English-language digital document images and when tested for Indian languages like Telugu they have failed to produce good results. This may be due to the complexity involved with the Telugu word images. An efficient algorithm was not devised till now that can extract Telugu word images accurately. Further, Telugu word image retrieval (TWIR) with the noisy, occlusion-affected and random

DOI: 10.1201/9781003132110-9

distorted query words has not been discussed in the recent literature. Furthermore, TWIR is a difficult and challenging task due to the fact that each word image has its own structure with a single and multi-conjunct vowel-consonant cluster. Hence, to retrieve those types of word images, one must obtain the most effective features that describe the relevant data of query Telugu word images even in the case of all possible distortions. Another important area that has not been investigated is the retrieval of multi-conjunct vowel-consonant clustered word images with missing word segments from the Telugu word images. To achieve this, an efficient feature extraction algorithm can be developed which can exact the most relevant features that describe the relevant data. Then the effective features can be utilised to retrieve the desired information even in the presence of all types of possible degradations like missing segments, noise, corrupted and occlusion-affected word images and multi-conjunct vowel-consonant clustered word images. This motivates us to develop a high-level feature extraction for a TWIR system for Telugu word images.

Image retrieval [2] has been broadly classified into two types, namely text-based approach and content-based approach. Each approach has its own unique features [3] that can be used in various applications based on their scenario. Content-based image retrieval (CBIR) [4] is also known as query by image content. With this approach the search analyses the visual content of the image rather than keyword descriptions associated with the image [5]. Text-based image retrieval (TBIR) [6] is purely based on text keyword descriptions used as input and index images also using text keywords. By comparing both input keywords and index image keywords, the matching images are retrieved from the image repository. The advantages of this approach are ease of implementation, fast retrieval and Web image search. The most ideal method for handling these digital archives is to segment the text present in the image documents. Once the segmentation of text is done, an efficient representational method (profile feature) can be applied to get the segmented data in the representation form which can be useful for a content-based image retrieval system. Another way of handling this is to use a direct method that converts the digital documents into text by optical character recognisers (OCRs). OCR recognises the text from the document images. The efficiency of OCR use defines the performance of the OCR-based text-image retrieval scheme. As per the available literature, the utilisation and use of OCR frameworks are defined and applied to different languages around the world. The OCRs are commercially available for a few Oriental scripts and Latin languages. India is a diversified country where different languages are spoken in different states. The literature explains that there is less focus on the development of robust OCRs for the Indian languages. Numerous techniques were developed by the researchers to extract text from the digital documents based on the language considered. Disadvantages are that annotation of images manually is not available most of the time; annotation is difficult for a large image repository when manually annotated; and manual annotation is not accurate [7]. The expected visual content or image is not exactly retrieved by the user through a query and the second one refers to the difficulty in relating high-level semantic concepts with low-level visual features. In order to overcome these two challenges, researchers have focused their efforts on the TWIR systems [8]. With this approach visual content plays a major role in the retrieval of word images such as texture, colour, intensity, shape, resolution, etc. [9]. At present, the scenario image retrieval domain has faced lots of challenges [10] due to its growth of digitisation in day-to-day activities. Though there are diverse kinds of word and grammar issues in the script domain, symbol density issues are one of the major problems. To manage such symbol issues, proposed TWIR informatics repositories play an important role. Digitisation of files has opened several opportunities in imparting sizeable entry of data and growing information for constructing language processing pipelines including system translation and search engines. These digitised files are both scanned, published or handwritten, and consist of books, manuscripts, letters, invoices, catalogues, etc. Content-degree that gets entry to this substantial virtual corpus is viable. Given the advancements in the field of word image retrieval (WIR), one can build robust and innovative solutions using the information produced from an ideal recogniser. However, an optical character recogniser (OCR) recognises only the individual character, and still, it must mature since OCR is not suitable for the retrieval of word images that are scanned and degraded, which is an efficient approach these days over the single-character recognition using OCR [1]. This leads us to the approach which can be considered as a complementary method where the idea is to formulate the problem from a "retrieval" perspective. In this setting, given a query word image, one must rank all word images from the candidate set in the order of its similarity. Here both the query and word images from the database are represented using a holistic representation that captures the lexical information of the word in feature space. The design of these holistic representations is one of the major challenges to be solved, which decides the effectiveness of Telugu script image retrieval methods.

The words in document images are represented by a set of features. Usually, features are vectors of numeric values. The features used for representing the objects in different applications may differ for similar objects. The change in the feature values would be due to a change in the appearance of the objects or the viewing angle. Even in document images, the appearance of words may change due to several factors that arise at the time of digitisation. The print style of the documents and the type of font also affect the representation. The representation of similar words printed in different fonts varies considerably. The search within a collection of words involves looking for similar words [2, 3]. The simple solution is to match the query word image with all the words in the collection and report similar ones. Direct matching of image pixels may fail even in the presence of small changes in the sizes of images [4]. Moreover, there will be several variations occurring in words due to artefacts, digitisation process and size changes, etc. [5, 6]. Searching for similar words in a collection is challenging. However, many methods have overcome this problem with the invention of new techniques. The word images are represented by a set of features [7], usually vectors or sequences of numeric values. These representations are used for word image matching. Thus, similar words can be searched using the matching technique. A similarity measure that looks for approximate matches, to some extent, may be one of the methods for image matching. This method of searching similar words by image matching technique is expensive. As a result of matching the query with every word of the collection, the search may take more time to generate the results. Hence, exhaustive search techniques are not suitable for searching in word image collections.

The major contribution of the proposed methodology is as follows:

- Initially, all the images are normalised to the fixed size, so all the train and test image features will be perfectly estimated. This normalisation process is also used to calculate and analyse the various distortions such as missing segment with distortion, random distortion, noise effect and missing segment in query words.
- The DLCNN approach is applied to extract both textural and static features from Telugu words. The major significance of DLCNN is to analyse word images and analysis them with respect to Telugu symbols.
- Then, the DeepCluster process is applied to the feature vectors by using the AlexNet deep learning model. Thus, here input features will be divided into various classes based on their grammatical significance and rules.
- Finally, pairwise Hamming distance measurement is used to compare the various features within the database along with its classes and retrieves the similar resultant output images based on their indexes.
- The proposed results are compared to the various litterers such as SDM-NSCT [11], HWNET v2 [12], GLCM-IPC [13], SURF-BoVW [14], HMM-C [15] and SIFT-BoVW [16] and provide better precision and recall accuracy.

The rest of the chapter is organised as follows: Section 9.2 gives the detailed explanation of various state-of-the-art approaches with their drawbacks. Section 9.3 gives the detailed procedure of the proposed TWIR system using training and testing phases with DLCNN-based feature extraction and DeepCluster-based feature clustering. Section 9.4 gives the analysis of the simulation results of the proposed approach and compares it with the existing methods. Finally, future enhancements are shown in Section 9.5.

9.2   REVIEW OF LITERATURE

Due to the advancements and technologies to the digital industry, scanned old documents have been preserved using digital libraries and are available in the digital archives electronically. Improper digital scanning and storage may occur during the scanning of some documents. High rates of errors may result in these document images owing to factors like folding, occlusion, random noise, cut type, etc. A better manual or automatic searching mechanism requires searching the degraded scanned documents from the collections. The possible solution would be automatic and efficient search strategies for enhanced performance of image search engines instead of manual searching which is time-consuming and more expensive computationally. The searching and retrieval of degraded Telugu documents are focused on in this research work based on word images as keywords. From collections of document images, highly degraded document image retrieval has been considered. Features are extracted from the provided trained images and query word images in keyword searching. According to the feature distance, the matching is performed. In keyword searching, major challenges include feature comparison mechanism selection and robust features extraction.

In this chapter, the WIR with recent methodologies is reviewed and we fill in the gaps in regard to several relevant works. We have examined and addressed the challenges and nature of texts using WIR methods. Based on the relevant feedback, the retrieval enhancement methods have been utilised after completing the core steps that contain the WIR system and the obtained results will improve. For analysing the performance, the evaluation standards and measures have been demonstrated, and the results of state-of-the-art methods have been investigated. A challenging issue is the related word images' retrieval from a database of word images. For this problem, three dimensions have been included, such as 1) how to match or compare the representations of two word images, 2) how to represent the word images and 3) how to retrieve accurately and efficiently if the database size grows.

If there is a text representation, all these problems are relatively easier if it can be obtained based on an OCR system. The robust and reliable OCR systems are not available for the Telugu language [1]. These are digitised and archived but the complete content level access is not available for the collection. To recognise the free retrieval, WIR [5] has become an emergent solution. By using a distance parameter, the representation of word images and comparison have been performed with some features. Word spotting has the benefit of not requiring prior learning owing to the nature of appearance-based matching. In TWIR, such schemes of word matching have been utilised popularly. In the previous studies, various research has been performed that focuses on different problems such as different embedding methods, data modality (printed, scene text and handwritten) and representation nature, either variable length or fixed. The more robust representations have resulted in the recent proliferation of deep learning methods into the document community. The related words are categorised into three phases such as (1) establishment of classical techniques based on the representation of variable length, (2) representation of fixed length achieved with the bag of words framework and (3) building of learned representation through various classifier models and deep learning networks on the top of hand-crafted features.

Later, Sekhar et al. presented an efficient and accurate word image retrieval using the BoVW approach from a large database [17]. This approach is highly scalable and language independent. They also showed that a text retrieval system can be adapted to build a word image retrieval solution, which helped in obtaining scalability. Four Indian languages have been utilised in this work. Further, they also described their future enhancements towards the word image retrieval system. One group [16] applied bag of visual words (BoVW) features for word image retrieval by refining classification accuracy using fused SIFT and BoVW textural features. This work outperforms normal word images classification by using fused LBP and BoVW features. This feature gave more accurate results when compared to other image features. But again, there are more features available to enhance the classification accuracy for an effective image retrieval system. Textural feature extraction based on a hidden Markov model (HMM) on the printed Telugu documents has been proposed [15].

To improve the performance they used HMM-based coarseness textural features. The feature extraction of the HMM model is degraded due to it not supporting the statistical features, hence reducing the retrieval accuracy.

One group of authors [14] proposed a retrieval system using SURF feature extraction along with the BoVW model. With this paper, the authors have studied the use of a SURF + BoVW model to improve the digital word images for classifying various problems in script readings. SURF is more suitable for extracting image features like bright or dark in both backgrounds and foregrounds of the image. With this justification, the work has been developed and results also improved a certain amount. The challenges of classifying word images are still motivated among researchers and academicians due to the size of images. But this method results in low precision values. Another group of authors [13] proposed the TWIR system using iterative portion clustering (IPC) of Telugu word data and grey level co-occurrence matrix (GLCM)-based feature extraction which results in reduced retrieval efficiency. A word image retrieval by texture characterisation by an HWNET v2–based deep learning system has been proposed [12]. But this deep learning model has high computational complexity resulting in more training and testing time compared to other approaches. This group [11] implemented the TWIR system using SDM-based NSCT feature extraction. Here deep convolution neural network is used for classifying Telugu word images and during training, it learned features and the classification results are used to retrieve word images. But this system gives less accuracy towards the various distortions and noises. In another proposal, a heterogeneity-aware multi-resolution local binary pattern (hmLBP) for retrieval of histopathology images [18]. Initially, in hmLBP, texture features were extracted from different resolutions of histology images and texture features were combined which acted as a final feature vector. Then, rotation invariant binary codes were used to extract compact binary codes. It reduced the dimensionality of the feature vector and comprised the vast majority of texture patterns. Finally, the histogram bins were weighted through counted LBP codes. However, it has a low F1 measure.

One group supplied more than one classifier for colour photo retrieval and the usage of a location-developing method [19]. They proposed artificial capabilities to explain the indoor shape and worldwide form for trademark photo retrieval. They mixed form description and characteristic matching to retrieve trademark photos. While another group [20] supplied an integration of worldwide-nearby descriptors to extract the capabilities via Zernike moment's coefficients and facet gradient coincidence matrix. To enhance the overall performance of TIR, we've used entropy as a refinement layer to cast off the distinct trademark photos after which we implemented Zernike moments and a SURF characteristic descriptor to retrieve maximum comparable photos.

There are a number of word-recognising applications for file indexing and retrieval which include the following:

- Retrieval of files with a given phrase in organisation files.
- Looking online in cultural historical past collections saved in libraries all around the world.

- Computerised sorting of handwritten mail containing significant words (e.g. "urgent", "cancelation", "complain").
- Identification of figures and their corresponding captions.
- Keyword retrieval in pre-health facility care reports (PCR forms).
- Word recognising in graphical files along with maps.
- Retrieval of cuneiform systems from historic clay tablets.
- Assisting human transcribers in figuring out words in degraded files, mainly the ones appearing for the first time.

9.3 PROPOSED METHOD

The main idea of this work is to benefit from the powerful performance of DLCNN aiming to extract effective features while minimising time and resources. CNN is the convolutional phase that works like a visual descriptor to extract features from images. Each image undergoes a transformation through an application of a set of filters creating new forms of images called convolution maps. These convolution maps are concatenated into a feature vector called CNN code. All features are saved as an index of features. This process has a training phase that is intended to extract the features from the dataset's images and a test phase that is used to extract features from the query. Our approach takes place in two phases and is represented in Figure 9.1.

For the retrieval process, a similarity comparison technique has been used between a test user query image and the training classified image feature database. After comparison, the resulting images are identified and retrieved based on their shortest distance. The shortest-distance image between the query image and the classified image feature database will be considered as the first-ranked image for the best match retrieval.

- *Training phase*: In this phase, the features are extracted from the dataset using DLCNN, and then the component analysis–based DeepCluster clustering algorithm is used to cluster images into similar groups and determine the gravity centre of each group. The gravity centres construct the output layer in the retrieving phase and will be used as an identifier for each group.
- *Test phase*: In this phase, the similarity between features extracted from a query using DLCNN and the output layer of a CNN to predict the identifier closer to it is calculated. Based on that calculation, the closest cluster is returned. Then, when the similarity is calculated between the query and the images in that cluster, the top-ranking images are finally retrieved.

9.3.1 NORMALISATION OF THE IMAGES

For image normalisation, all the random-sized images are resized into same-sized images to extract multiple features of the image on the same structure. Here the random-sized images are normalised as 200×400-size pixel images without affecting the aspect ratio of the image using bilinear standard transformation. This normalisation process is also used to calculate and analyse the various distortions such

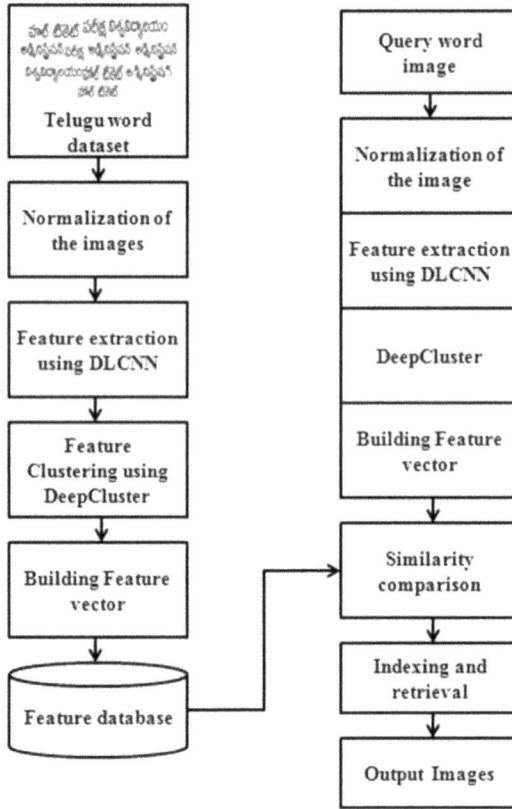

FIGURE 9.1 Proposed TWIR model.

as missing segment with distortion, random distortion, noise effects and missing segment in query words.

9.3.2 FEATURE EXTRACTION USING DLCNN

For feature extraction, the most popular deep learning algorithm called DLCNN has been used. A CNN is a neural network process which changes a function into some other form to get more details of the image by performing the element-wise matrix multiplication operation between the original image and the filter or kernel image. Here DLCNN is used for extracting Telugu word image features such as shape and texture since Telugu word images are in a different shape and texture format.

Figure 9.2 shows the proposed DLCNN model for the extraction of features. In convolution operations, there are two matrixes of which one is an image matrix and the other is a filter or kernel matrix that transforms the image into another format. The transformed images are called convoluted images. In this work normalised Telugu word image matrixes are given as input to the convolution neural network to

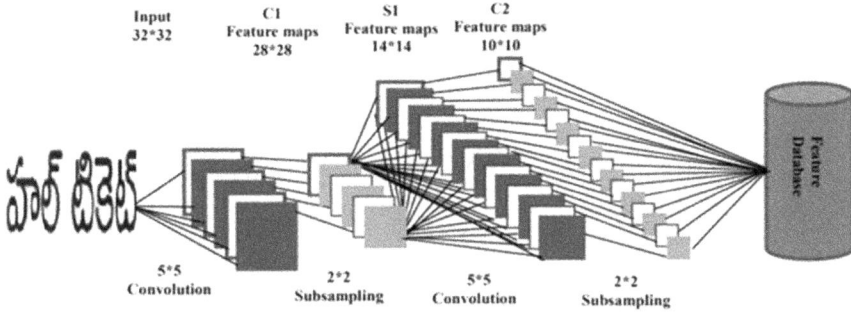

FIGURE 9.2 The process of convolution for feature extraction.

convert a convoluted image matrix from where features are extracted to build a feature vector for the retrieval process. The sample Telugu word input image matrix and corresponding convoluted image matrix us CNN filter or kernel. As we have used 5 × 5 matrixes for the input image, for this example total pixels points are 25. After applying convolution computation that has been reduced as 9-point pixels since that convolution filter or kernel has 3 × 3. This process has been applied until the fine details of features are extracted.

The entire process of convolution starts from raw Telugu word images and builds them into feature vectors for the retrieval process. Here we have used 32 × 32 × 1 images for the entire convolution process. Firstly, 5 × 5 kernels with one stride are used over a 32 × 32 × 1 image as the convolution layer and a 28 × 28 × 6 output matrix is generated. The feature map is reduced as 28 × 28 from 32 × 32 with one stride and no padding. Secondly, an average pooling method has been used for dimension reduction. For dimension reduction, we have used a filter size of 2 × 2 with a stride of 2 and the dimension was reduced by the factor of 2. This would yield a 14 × 14 × 6. Likewise, another convolution layer was used with 16 5 × 5 kernels to get an output matrix of 10 × 10 × 6. Subsequently, another pooling layer was used that yielded an output matrix of 5 × 5 × 16. Finally, 16 5 × 5 feature maps were extracted from each image and each feature maps consist of a width of 5 × 5 matrixes. In this work, the fully connected layers in the pre-trained DLCNN models are excluded from the network. That means only the convolutional layers remained in the model for features extraction. The advantage of using those pre-trained images is that they have learned to extract features from a diversity of images. The signature of each Telugu word image was represented by a vector that includes features extracted from the DLCNN model. Then, based on those signatures, we cluster the images.

9.3.3 Feature Clustering

In this section, the proposed DeepCluster is proposed for the cluttering of features. The convolution layers and pooling layers extract the textual features and image features. Then extracted features are processed in the clustering layer which is introduced in the fully connected layer. It takes advantage of the high capacity of an

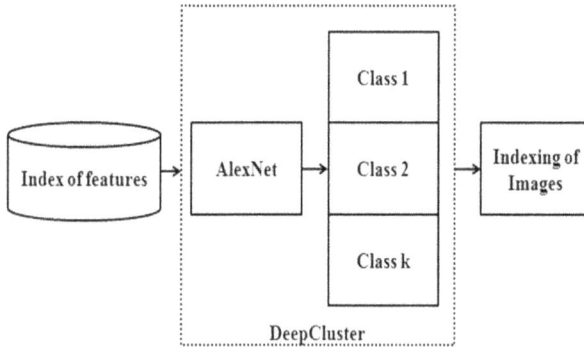

FIGURE 9.3 DeepCluster approach.

optimised AlexNet and the ability to learn the clusters without labels. The cluster labels are used in the fully connected layer to classify the images as relevant and non-relevant images. The relevant images are ranked based on the minimum distance between relevant images and the database images. Figure 9.3 shows the overall flow of this DeepCluster method.

The textual description and the collected images are given as input to the optimised AlexNet. The convolution layer and pooling layer are processed to extract the textual features and visual features. In the classification task, an optimised AlexNet aims to generate predictions from a labelled dataset. By learning this mapping using the optimised AlexNet, the measurement of the data area is decreased to a much smaller area with the assistance of max-ave pooling layers and completely convolutional layers. The optimised AlexNet summarises the functions of textual facts of the images and visible images. As a result, every layer of optimised AlexNet may be interpreted as a function embedding of the data.

Generally, a set of clustering rules organises an unlabeled dataset into clusters. The clustering set of rules has the advantage of being capable of generating clusters immediately from the data with no labels. The clustering set of rules plays higher because the size of the data area is reduced. The main intention of DeepCluster is to combine the optimised AlexNet and clustering process for efficient TWIR. In the deeply embedded clustering, optimised AlexNet learns mapping between the textual information of images and visual images in the dataset to the query. The embedded clustering technique groups the images into different categories from lower-dimensional embedding. The optimised AlexNet consists of five convolution layers, three pooling layers and three fully connected layers. The convolutional and pooling layer is used to extract the textual features and visual features of images. The DeepCluster is designed such that the second fully connected layer of optimised AlexNet acts as an embedded clustering layer. It is a fully connected layer without max-out activation, with the number of units equal to the number of classes of the dataset. The embedded clustering layer uses a t-distribution kernel to measure the similarity between embedding textual and visual features of images and the mean of a cluster distribution.

The probability of an image belonging to a cluster is the embedding textual and visual features of images and is the hyper-parameter. The first fully connected convolutional layer extracts the global features of textual visual information of images. The second fully connected layer of optimised AlexNet learns the centroids of different clusters representing each class. This layer is used to learn the mapping between the embedding textual and visual features of images and the predictions. Moreover, the frequencies are designed to prevent distortion from massive clusters. A Kullback-Leibler divergence is computed as a loss characteristics to examine the goal photo and embed possibility distributions. For the clustering layer, the loss is related to the cluster centres and the embedding of textual and visible functions of images. The cluster centre (i.e. centroid) with minimum loss is used for further process.

9.3.3.1   Indexing of Images

The centroids of each cluster are used as a class label which is given as input to the next layer. It maps the cluster labels with the relevant images by using an activation function. The sigmoid logistic regression function controls the output between the cluster labels obtained from the clustering layer, which are the weights in this layer and the bias in the last fully connected layer. Then the binary operation is performed where the feature vectors of the relevant images are mapped into binary codes. After the classification of images, relevant images are ranked based on the pairwise Hamming distance of binary codes between relevant images and database images.

9.3.4   Retrieving Images Using DLCNN

The retrieving phase is a test and requires a pairwise Hamming distance measure to search for similar images. First, the DLCNN node (already stored as small signature files) from the query is compared to the output layer of the convolution phase. The comparison is taken based on their pairwise Hamming similarity scores between the features. The closest centroid to the query represents the identifier of the relevant class. Finally, we retrieve the top images from the selected cluster. The relevant image which has minimum pairwise Hamming distance has the topmost rank.

9.4   RESULTS AND DISCUSSION

This section gives a detailed analysis of simulation results of the proposed system implemented using a MATLAB 2019a programming environment. To effectively implement the proposed system, standard books are considered from various Indian digital libraries such as the Digital Library of India and the Universal Library, respectively. The proposed system trained with the various types of books obtained from these libraries. Table 9.2 presents the various types of Telugu books such as novels, arts, commerce, history, philosophy, psychology, engineering, architecture, mythology and so on considered for the training process with the available pages and words. Nearly one million words overall are used for the training procedure.

Figure 9.4 gives the sample test Telugu word images with various grammars and distortions. The distortions are a missing segment with distortion, a random distortion,

TABLE 9.1
Proposed TWIR Procedure

Step 1: Load the image from the database.

Step 2: Extract local features of both textual and visual information of images by processing convolutional layer and max-pooling layer.

Step 3: Extract global features of both textual and visual information of images by processing first fully connected layer.

Step 4: Cluster the features by processing the clustering layer.

Step 5: Classify the images as relevant and non-relevant images based on the cluster labels by processing the hidden layer.

Step 6: Map the relevant image with the binary codes by performing binary operation.

Step 7: Calculate the pairwise Hamming distance between the relevant images and database images and rank the images based on the pairwise Hamming distance.

TABLE 9.2
Book Used for Experiment

Telugu Book Type	No. of Books	Average Pages per Book	Total Words
History and mythology	2	200	22,048
Arts and commerce	3	350	32,038
Telugu literature	7	280	37,501
Science and technology	7	300	64,993

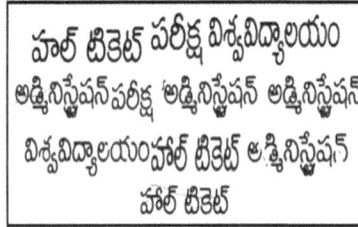

FIGURE 9.4   Test images utilised for TWIR system.

noise effects and a missing segment. These distortions are generated due to various noise sources, typing mistakes caused by humans or machine printing and scanning problems. Thus it is necessary to analyse the performance of the proposed system using precision and recall metrics. For analysing the performance of the proposed TWIR system, mAR and mAP metrics are calculated and compared with the state-of-the-art approaches. They are SDM-NSCT [11], HWNET v2 [12], GLCM-IPC [13], SURF-BoVW [14], HMM-C [15] and SIFT-BoVW [16]. The proposed simulation is performed by using various types of test images and gives the enhancive mAP and mAR because the proposed method utilises the advanced deep learning architectures for feature extraction and feature clustering based on the grammatical rules.

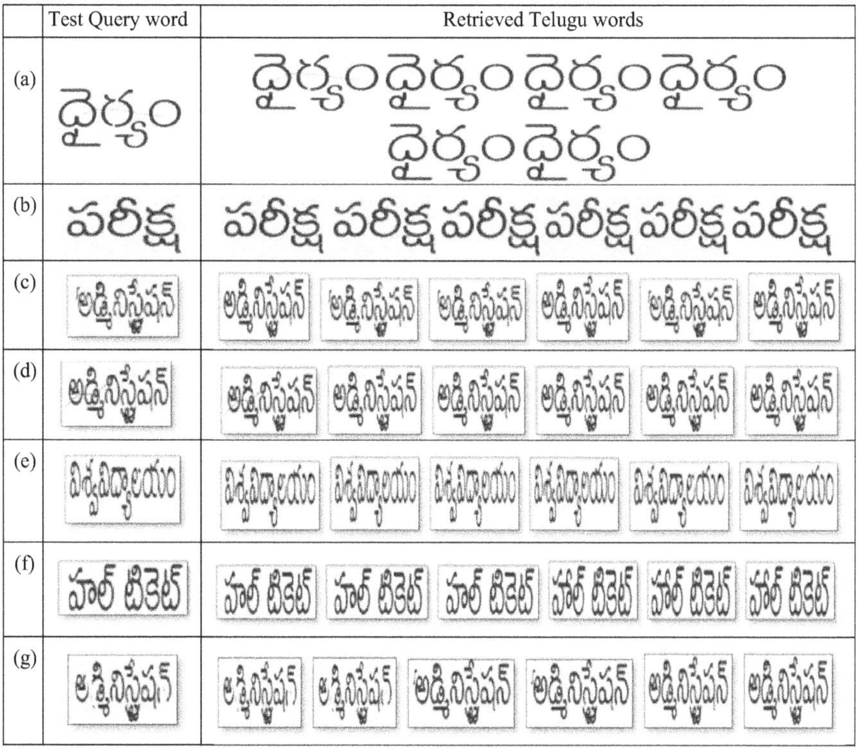

FIGURE 9.5 Retrieved output Telugu word images with DLCNN and DeepCluster. (a) Missing segment with random distortion, (b) noisy as a query word, (c) occlusion effected, (d) random disturbance and (e), (f), (g) missing segment words.

Figure 9.5 represents the retrieved output Telugu word images for various query words with distortions. Column two represents the all-query word images whereas column three represents the retrieved word images for that query word. Figure 9.5a, e, f and g represent the scenario of retrieved images for a missing segment with random distortion and missing segment words-based query images. Even though some parts of Telugu symbols are missed, by using deep feature clustering output, images are retrieved very precisely. Figure 9.5d represents the scenario of retrieved images for random disturbance-based query images. Even though lots of disturbances occurred in both trained and testing images, by using DLCNN feature learning with normalisation output images are retrieved very precisely. Figure 9.5c represents the scenario of retrieved images for occlusion-affected query images. Here, extra unintended and unwanted occlusion lines are drawn on both trained and testing images, and by using DLCNN feature learning with normalisation output images are retrieved accurately. And finally, Figure 9.5b represents the scenario of retrieved images for noise-affected query images. Here, the proposed deep learning approach by default eliminates all types of noise and improves retrieval accuracy.

TABLE 9.3

Performance Comparison of Proposed TWIR with Existing Systems

Measurement	SIFT + BoVW [16]	HMM-C [15]	SURF+ BoVW [14]	GLCM-IPC [13]	HWNET v2 [12]	SDM-NSCT [11]	Proposed TWIR System
mAP	0.853	0.89	0.731	0.967	0.978	0.998	0.999
mAR	0.799	0.823	0.809	0.842	0.92	0.98	0.999

Table 9.3 represents the performance comparison of the proposed TWIR system using deep learning–based feature extraction and feature clustering with the various literature. From Table 9.3 the simulation results show the superior performance of mAP and mAR metrics compared to SDM-NSCT [11], HWNET v2 [12], GLCM-IPC [13], SURF-BoVW [14], HMM-C [15] and SIFT-BoVW [16], respectively.

9.5 CONCLUSION

This work presents the efficient mechanism of the TWIR system using deep learning–based feature extraction and feature clustering approaches. Initially, the normalisation process was applied, so all the test and training image sizes are perfectly adjusted to an equal level. It helped to extract justified texture features with reduced losses and distortions. Then, DLCNN architecture was applied to extract all types of word features based on the Telugu alphabet modelling. Then, an AlexNet-based DeepCluster method was applied for effectively analysing the words and classifying the features based on the Telugu grammar, thus words were indexed based on features with their grammatical attributes. Finally, pairwise Hamming distance was utilised to find the similarity between query words and the database. The simulations were performed against various distortion scenarios such as missing segments with distortion, random distortion, noise effects and missing segmentst in query words. And in all those scenarios, the proposed TWIR method gives the better mAP and mAR performance evaluation compared to existing methods. This work can be extended to implement a real-time word search assistance system for Indian digital libraries by incorporating all the Indian languages.

REFERENCES

1. Li, Ang, et al. "Generating holistic 3D scene abstractions for text-based image retrieval." In *Proceedings of the IEEE Conference on Computer Vision and Pattern Recognition* (2017).
2. Unar, Salahuddin, et al. "Detected text-based image retrieval approach for textual images." *IET Image Processing* 13.3 (2019): 515–521.
3. MK, Yanti Idaya Aspura, and Shahrul Azman Mohd Noah. "Semantic text-based image retrieval with multi-modality ontology and DBpedia." *The Electronic Library* (2017).
4. Zeng, Mengqi, et al. "CATIRI: An efficient method for content-and-text based image retrieval." *Journal of Computer Science and Technology* 34.2 (2019): 287–304.
5. Parcalabescu, Letitia, and Anette Frank. "Exploring phrase grounding without training: Contextualisation and extension to text-based image retrieval." In *Proceedings of the IEEE/CVF Conference on Computer Vision and Pattern Recognition Workshops* (2020).
6. Estrela, Vania Vieira, and Albany E. Herrmann. "Content-based image retrieval (CBIR) in remote clinical diagnosis and healthcare." In *Encyclopedia of E-Health and Telemedicine*. IGI Global (2016): 495–520.
7. Zaidi, Syed Ali Jafar, et al. "Implementation and comparison of text-based image retrieval schemes." *International Journal of Advanced Computer Science and Applications* 10.1 (2019): 611–618.

8. Unar, Salahuddin, et al. "A decisive content based image retrieval approach for feature fusion in visual and textual images." *Knowledge-Based Systems* 179 (2019): 8–20.

9. Zhou, Wengang, Houqiang Li, and Qi Tian. "Recent advance in content-based image retrieval: A literature survey." *arXiv preprint arXiv:1706.06064* (2017).

10. Hossain, M. S., and Islam, M. R.. "A new approach of content based image retrieval using color and texture features." *Current Journal of Applied Science and Technology* 21.3 (2017): 1–16. https://doi.org/10.9734/BJAST/2017/33326.

11. Lakshmi, K. M., and T. R. Babu. "Robust algorithm for Telugu word image retrieval and recognition." *Journal of Mechanics of Continua and Mathematical Sciences* 14.1 (2019).

12. Krishnaann, P., and C. V. Jawahaar. "HWNET v2: An efficient word image representation for handwritten documents." *Computer Vision and Pattern Recognition* (2018).

13. Lakshmi, K. M., and T. R. Babu. "A new hybrid algorithm for telugu word retrieval and recognition." *International Journal of International Education Studies* 11.4 (2018): 117–127.

14. Jayanthi, N., and S. Indhu. "Inscription IR using bag-of-visual words." *IOP Conference Series: MSE* 225.1 (2017): 1–8.

15. Nagasudhha, D., and Y. M. Lattha. "Keyword spotting using HMM in trinted Telugu documents." In *Proceedings of International Conference on SCOPES*, Paralakhemundi, India (2016): 1997–2000.

16. Shekhar, R., and C. V. Jawahar. "WIR using bag of visual words." In *IAPS International Workshop on DAS*, Gold Cost, QLD (2012): 297–301.

17. Shekhar, R., and C. V. Jawahar. "Word image retrieval using bag of visual words." In *Proceedings of 10th IAPR International Workshop on Document Analysis* (2012).

18. Lakshmi, K. Mohana, and T. RangaBabu. "A novel Telugu script recognition and retrieval approach based on hash coded hamming." In *International Conference on Communications and Cyber Physical Engineering 2018*. Springer, Singapore (2018).

19. Pala, Mythilisharan, Laxminarayana Parayitam, and Venkataramana Appala. "Real-time transcription, keyword spotting, archival and retrieval for telugu TV news using ASR." *International Journal of Speech Technology* 22.2 (2019): 433–439.

20. Cheekati, Bindu Madhuri, and Roje Spandana Rajeti. "Telugu handwritten character recognition using deep residual learning." In *2020 Fourth International Conference on I-SMAC (IoT in Social, Mobile, Analytics and Cloud)(I-SMAC)*. IEEE (2020).

10 Smart Health Informatics Systems

S. Vani, R. Srivel, G. Aparna and Palvadi Srinivas Kumar

CONTENTS

DOI: 10.1201/9781003132110-10

10.1 INTRODUCTION

10.1.1 GENERAL INTRODUCTION

The developed meaning of a robot can be characterised as an electro-mechanical gadget that adheres to a bunch of directions to do certain errands; however, in a real sense, "robot" implies a "slave". Robots discover wide applications, in businesses as industrial robots, in sci-fi films and in family errands as humanoids. Mechanical technology and computerisation can be very much accomplished in the event that we consolidate the two of them. Robots can perform undertakings naturally absent of a lot of human intercessions, aside from introductory programming and guidelines being given to them.

Robots are widely utilised in computerisation. The advanced mechanisms are increasing a lot; for example, they can change their position in various situations as needed.

The broader viewpoint on cutting-edge mechanics is actually the predictable endeavour of experts to make machines prepared for performing tasks as cautiously as humans can do, and moreover, the bewildering, outrageous and repetitive tasks that individuals would lean toward not doing. The types of progress in the field of mechanical innovation are the use of central processors and microcontrollers with the adroit blend of motors, sensors and actuators.

The degree of mechanical innovation has expanded and the robots which can simply deal with pre-altered rules autonomous of the conditions they are working in are after a short time going to get old. The robots cultivated these days can recognise their environmental factors and act similarly; considering their sensations of the environment, they settle on choices in isolation on to how to respond. Days are not far when robots will even identify and respond to conclusions and could even convey how they feel.

Fundamentally, the Pick and Place Multi-Axis Robotic Arm can be characterised in two sections:

- Programming
- Equipment

Both the parts are important to achieve the Pick and Place Multi-Axis Robotic Arm. The extent of this task will be centred on object arranging utilising a shading sensor. The extension will incorporate as follows:

- Utilise Arduino Mega 2560 and programming to mechanise the entire framework and legitimate testing.
- Plan and fabricate a transport constructed framework.

In addition, Pick and Place Multi-Axis Robotic Arm has a wide variety of uses in the field of instruction, investigation and electrical portability and so forth.

10.1.2   TYPES OF ROBOTS AND THEIR CLASSIFICATION

Robots exist in various structures, shapes and sizes. Robots do not really need to look like machines that are displayed in motion pictures or anecdotal shows. Once in a while, robots are made to perform extremely basic errands like cleaning the house or pulling substantial materials and so on. What's more, there are a few robots, which have been created for clinical purposes that can do a medical procedure too under the direction of the specialist. The significant sorts of robots that different businesses use to accomplish their particular objectives are as follows.

10.1.2.1   Types of Industrial Robots

Robots, depending on the industry and based on their use in a particular field of application, can be broadly classified into:

- *Manual handling device*: An operator is required to operate this.
- *Fixed sequence robot*: This type of robot is configured to execute a sequential task in a cyclic manner, the flow is fixed and was non-programmable.
- *Variable sequence robot*: These share the same operation sequence as that of fixed-sequence robots but differ only on the ground.
- *Playback robot*: These types of devices follow up playback sequences automatically in a loop.
- *Numerical control robot*: They are also sequence-based robots with their terms.
- *Intelligent robot*: These robots are designed with the capability to sense their location.

10.1.2.2   Types Based on Application

Robots based on their application can be classified into seven major types:

1. Industrial robots
   These types of robots are generally used in the industrial environment for carrying out various operations such as lifting heavy components or for pick-and-place operations, etc.
2. Domestic robots
   Domestic robots, as the name suggests, can be used at home to perform daily house chores.

3. Surgical robots
   These robots are used in performing surgeries that can be controlled by doctors from a remote distance.
4. Robots used in space research programmes (robonauts)
   These robots are used in various space research programmes. They are multipurpose robots and can be both humanoid as well as non-humanoid.
5. Commercial entertainment robots
   These types of robots are generally used for entertainment purposes.
6. Army robots
   Robots that are used in defence fall into this category.
7. Service robots
   Service robots are those robots that are used in institutions or R&D teams to implement new features.

10.1.2.3 Types Based on Kinematics

1. Stationary robots: Stationary robots, as the name suggests, are a fixed type of robotic arm with a global axis of movement.
    (i) Cartesian robots: Robots with the capability to move in X-Y-Z coordinates fall under this category.
    (ii) Cylindrical robots: Robots with basic rotation capability. They can move in a linear and angular fashion.
    (iii) Spherical robots: This type of robot works in a spherical system.
    (iv) SCARA robots: This type of robot has a parallel-axis joint layout, the arm is slightly compliant in the X-Y direction but rigid in the Z direction.
    (v) Articulated robots: This robotic configuration is befitted with three revolute joints.
    (vi) Parallel robots: These are closed-loop systems to support a single platform. A classic example of this kind of robot is flight simulators.
2. Wheeled robots: These robots can be further classified as:
    (i) Single-wheel robots
    (ii) Two-wheel robots
    (iii) Three-or-more-wheel robots
3. Legged robots:
    (i) Bipedal robots (humanoid robots)
    (ii) Tri-pedal robots: Robots with three articulated limbs
    (iii) Quadrupedal robots
    (iv) Hexapod robots
4. Swimming robots
5. Flying robots

10.1.3 IMPORTANCE OF A MICROCONTROLLER

A microcontroller is a prototyping software wherein you can test out various circuits of your own ideas. It is based on the microcontroller ATmega328P of the

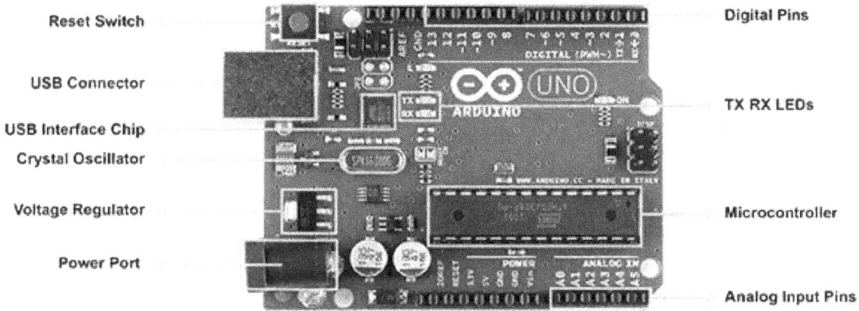

FIGURE 10.1 Parts of a microcontroller.

Atmel series. Basically it has its own CPU along with a control unit and ALU arithmetic and logic unit (for various mathematical operations) and memory. It has its own software (Arduino IDE) where you can work that is based on C language. It has various digital and analogue ports where you can play around with a lot of sensors (Figure 10.1).

- Power (USB/barrel jack)
- Pins (5V, 3.3V, GND, analogue, digital, PWM, AREF)
- Reset button
- Power LED indicator
- TX RX LEDs
- Main IC
- Voltage regulator

- Power (USB):
    Arduino boards can be powered directly from the AC mains power supply by connecting it to the barrel jack.
- Pins:
    Arduino UNO has 14 digital input/output pins (out of which six can be used as PWM outputs), six analogue input pins and a USB connection.
    There are three main pins which are:
  a. Analogue reference pin.
  b. Digital ground.
  c. Digital pins 2–13.
  d. Digital pins 0–1/serial in/out—TX/RX: these pins cannot be used for digital i/o (digitalRead and digitalWrite).
- Reset button:
    The reset button does pretty much the same as unplugging the board and plugging it back in. It restarts your programme from the beginning.
    Hardware reset buttons on PCs work by pulling the reset line on the CPU, which resets it and causes the computer to reboot. Unlike Ctrl+Alt+Del,

pressing the reset button causes the BIOS to perform the POST check bring this line LOW to reset the microcontroller.

- Power LED:

    It is the basic LED where the power is ON when the whole device is connected to power and it may be a USB or adapter. When the power is on, the green-coloured light in the Arduino will blink. LED is on when the pin is on the high mode and LED is off when the pin is in the off mode.

    The green LED is marked with ON and it indicates that the Arduino has power. The yellow LED is marked L and is just connected to pin 13. So when we keep pin 13 at HIGH the LED light is on. A short one will drain the power away so there is no power in the Arduino.

- TX RX LEDs:

    "RX" and "TX" show the states of the receive and transmit pins, respectively, and allow you to see when serial communication is taking place.

    TTL logic levels are used for serial communication on TX/RX pins. These pins should not be connected directly to an RS232 serial port since they run at +/– 12V and may cause damage to your Arduino board. It connects to the computer through USB and communicates on digital pins 0 (RX) and 1 (TX).

- Main IC:

    ATMEL is a well-known manufacturer of microcontrollers. Before you load a new programme from the Arduino IDE, you need to know what IC your board has.

- Voltage regulator:

    The 5v generated on the Arduino UNO board can be connected to the controller's 5v pin to increase the power as needed. Electrolytic capacitors and ceramic capacitors are the two types of capacitors.

10.1.3.1 Programming a Microcontroller

Microcontrollers can be programmed and a set of instructions can help in controlling the I/O pins. Programming a microcontroller is easy if one has knowledge of coding the PC.

One important point to be kept in mind is that when you are programming a microcontroller, you are directly interacting with the hardware.

A variety of microcontrollers support a wide range of languages, amongst those, C being the most prominent. Other languages like C, C++ and BASIC are also supported.

10.1.4 NEED FOR THE PROJECT

So many elderly people and bedridden people nowadays are dependent on others for help to bring them small things near them; they want to lead an independent life without disturbing others but it doesn't come true. To avoid this we got this idea by researching several research papers and vlogs, and we came to bring a device which will help bedridden patients and elderly people. With the help of this device, they can easily get necessary things like a medicine box or something with the help of the controller which will be controlled through mobile Bluetooth.

10.1.5 APPLICATIONS OF THE PROJECT

The biggest challenge upfront to us humans is the lack of time. Time plays an important role in everyone's life. In today's world, we are seeing so many old people who are in bed unable to do their work, and the people who take care of them are also decreasing slowly day by day. This is the motivation for bringing up a project that can let a patient do his own work independently.

10.2   LITERATURE REVIEW

Many robotic procedures already have been performed and have yielded good outcomes. Acubot is the title of this robot, which was mentioned in a paper by Dan Stoianovici, Kevin Cleary and others.

As per today's situation due to COVID-19, people are getting afraid to visit patients or bedridden people or to go near them to give them things they need. In this pandemic situation, we can use this type of pick-and-place robotic arm prototype model for people and patients who are bedridden.

We can use this pick-and-place robotic arm in hospitals also, where the robot follows the line in between the beds of the patients, mostly in general wards.

The time of COVID-19 is upon us. The central objective of these robots is to limit individual-to-individual connection all while saving tidiness, virtue and backing in clinics and related offices, like separated wards. The clinical experts and specialists in charge of treating the coronavirus pandemic will experience a hazardous condition accordingly. The essential objective of this undertaking is to underscore the significance of clinically advanced mechanics overall by utilising these applications in detached wards, with the goal that emergency clinic organisations may expand the utilisation of clinical robots for various operations on a mechanised premise. Regardless of telemedicine's prosperity, it would just be helpful under certain conditions. Robots are assuming a functioning part in the new accomplishments of Korean and Chinese clinics and wellbeing areas, without any disappointments and without the utilisation of any clinical innovation.

10.3   DESIGN AND IMPLEMENTATION

10.3.1 MECHANICAL DESIGN

- The mechanical design is carried out carefully considering all the tolerance values of the joint, the base and the medical purpose for various components of the robotic arm.
- The design was carried out keeping in mind all the factors and components and giving them the required set of space for their effective functioning. The dimensions used in the design are the real-time dimensions of the components.

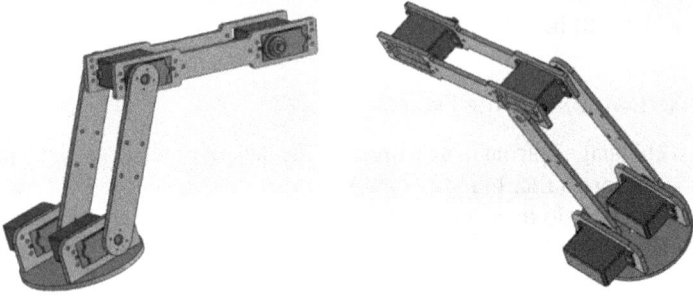

FIGURE 10.2   CAD model for robotic arm.

10.3.2   ROBOTIC ARM

- This type of robot is commonly used in modern manufacturing environments. These types of devices will perform all the given tasks (Figure 10.2).
- This is a three-axis robotic arm called the RRR manipulator. When compared to six-axis robotic arms, they typically have greater positioning accuracy.

10.3.3   MOTOR AND ITS POSITION

- There are two DC motors at the end joined to the base plate of the robotic arm (Figure 10.3).
- The simplest motors are DC motors. The rotational speed of a DC motor is determined by the input voltage if the DC motor receives a very high input voltage.

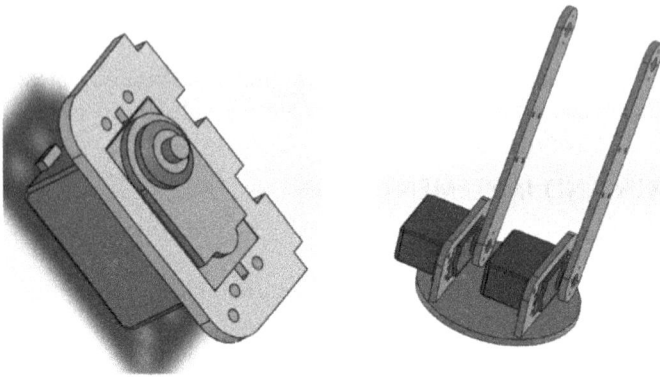

FIGURE 10.3   Motor and its position.

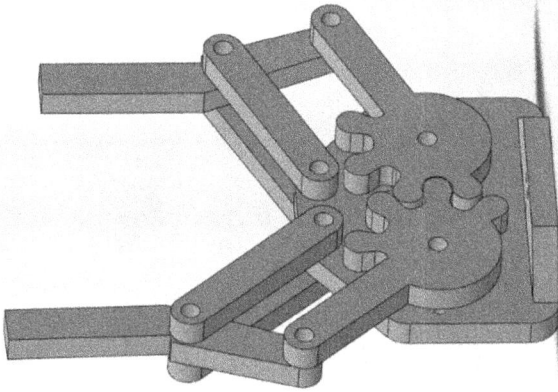

FIGURE 10.4   CAD model for the manipulator.

10.3.4 MANIPULATOR

The controller is the robot's whole instrument that permits it to move toward any path. The mobile segments of this automated controller are the joints, which permit relative movement between connecting joins. They additionally have an establishment, an arm and a gripper (Figure 10.4).

- This manipulator will help to pick and place the objects from one place to another place (Figures 10.5 and 10.6).

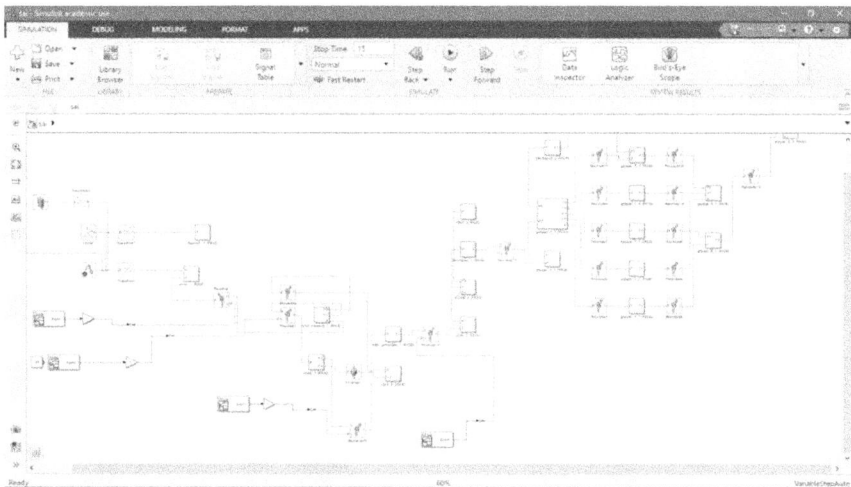

FIGURE 10.5   Simscape simulation.

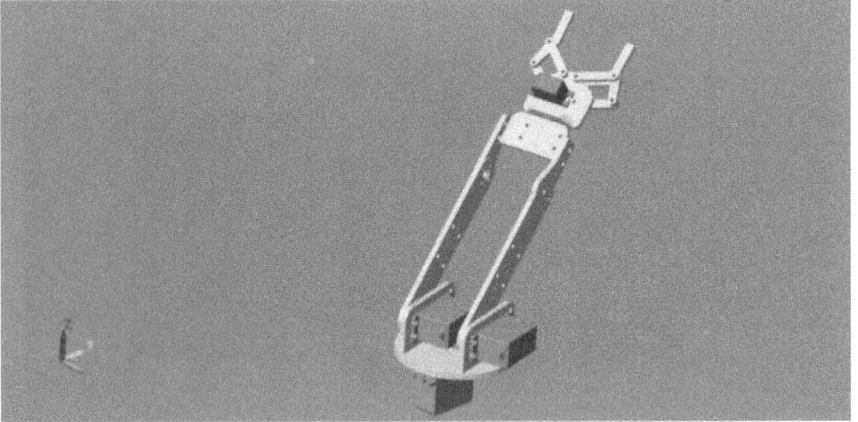

FIGURE 10.6 Screenshot of the MATLAB simulation.

- This model was developed in SolidWorks and, further, it was imported to the MATLAB using a SolidWorks MATLAB plugin.
- Upon importing, the joint was configured and the gravity was given in the z-axis.
- Later the ground was introduced to the environment.
- The robot is controlled by using angular controls so a Simulink-PS Converter is used to give the angular velocity inputs for the robot.

10.3.4.1 Electrical Components

To achieve the desired set of outputs, a system of motors, motor modules and an impeccable sensor system was brought into use. The components listed here comprise the electrical system.

- Arduino UNO
- NodeMCU
- IR sensors
- L293D motor driver
- Bluetooth
- Switch

10.3.4.2 Software Required

- Platform: Arduino IDE
- Programming language: Embedded C
- Four components needed

10.4 MOTORS

- According to the suggested name, it works on the direct current. It's a rotary device; in general, electrical motors are used to make the motion of the proposed system possible. They are the major part of the motion system of the project. A DC motor works on the principle of electromagnetic induction, where a conductor is put between a varying magnetic field or magnetic field is stationary and the conductor is brought into motion; due to these activities, an EMF or voltage gets produced. This principle is the driving force behind the DC motor operation.

• Although many variants of motors are available on the market, there were some reasons why the DC motor was opted for over any other contemporary motor.

10.4.1 ADVANTAGES

• Adequate speed control: By changing the armature or field voltage, a wide variation of speeds can be achieved, and also its controllability is high.
• Torque: The starting torque provided in DC motors is quite high, which makes it preferable in operations involving high load activities. Since they offer reconcilable drive power, that makes them also capable of holding constant torque.
• Smooth to operate: As the controllability varies over a wide range of speed variations these motors often provide a smooth and seamless operating experience.
• Avoidance of harmonics: DC motors are free from harmonics-related issues.

So keeping these points in consideration, we opted for DC motors. The motor used in the proposed system is a five-volt N20 motor (Figure 10.7).

Specifications of the motor used are listed below:

• Rated voltage: DC 5V
• No load current: 50 mA
• No load speed: 60 RPM
• Suitable voltage: DC (3–6)V
• Speed: 35 RPM–70 RPM
• Net weight: 10 g
• Rated torque: 2 Kg cm
• Material (gear): metallic

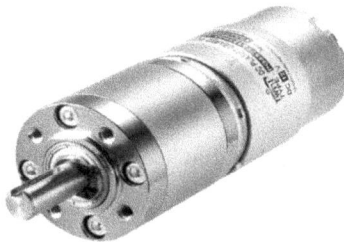

FIGURE 10.7 Motor.

- Total length: 34mm.
- Reduction ratio: 1:10.

10.4.2 Arduino UNO

- TUNO in Italian methods one, Arduino is an extraordinary instrument for creating intelligent models including sensors, controlling engines and different yields, and they can be associated with PC utilising USB [1].

10.4.2.1 Advantages

The biggest advantage of Arduino is it comes in a ready-to-use package, it contains oscillators, IR sensors and serial communication interface and headers. Another advantage is that its library of projects is present inside Arduino software, and Arduino also has automatic unit conversion capability [2].

10.4.2.2 Specifications

- Microcontroller: ATmega328P
- Operating voltage: 5v
- Input voltage: 7-20v
- Digital I/O pins: 14
- Analog input pins: 6
- DC Current per I/O; pin: 20 mA
- DC current for 3.3V; pin: 50 mA
- Flash memory: 32 KB, of which 0.5 KB is used by the bootloader
- SRAM: 2 KB
- EEPROM: 1 KB
- Clock speed: 16 MHz
- Length: 68.6 mm
- Width: 53.4 mm
- Weight: 25 g

10.4.3 Pin Configuration

1. Power USB: The Arduino board gets the power with a USB cable.
2. Power (barrel jack): The Arduino board can also be connected to the AC main power [3].
3. Voltage regulator: It regulates the voltage which is given to the Arduino UNO board.
4. Crystal oscillator: It deals with time-related issues, namely how Arduino calculates time.

Arduino reset 5 and 17 pins: The Arduino board can now receive a receipt through this section [4].

1. Press the number 17 to restart the computer.
2. An extra switch on pin 5 can be used to reset it.

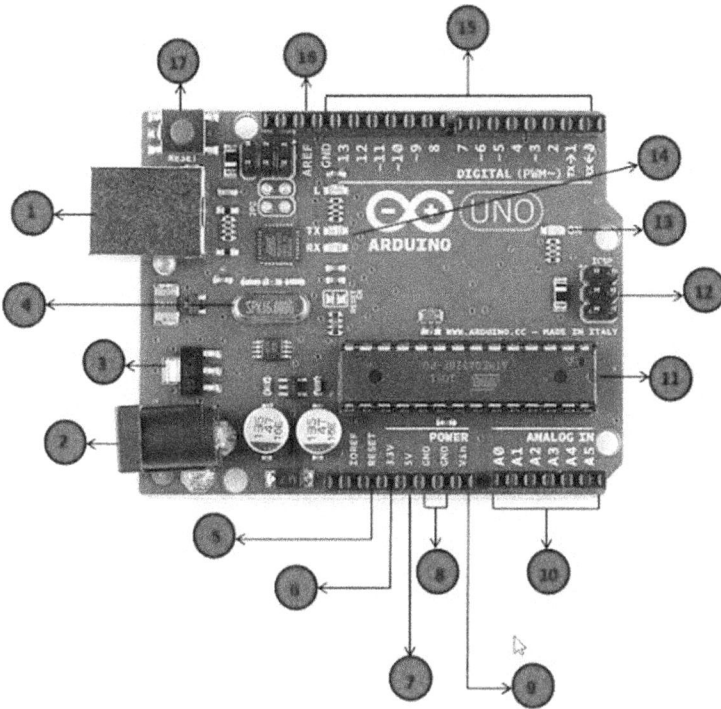

FIGURE 10.8   Arduino UNO microcontroller.

Pin 6,7,8,9:

Pin 6-3.3V: supplies 3.3-volt output.

Pin 7-5V: supplies 5-volt output.

Pin 8-GND (ground): there are a few ground pins on the Arduino.

Pin 9 vin: the ninth pin also can be used to give the power for the Arduino.

Analog PIN (10): There are five analogue input pins on the Arduino UNO, ranging from AO to A5.

The main microcontroller (11), also known as the Arduino board's brain, is found on each Arduino board. Arduino is a microcontroller.

Power LED indicator (13): with the power of the Arduino, the LED lights will be lit.

TX and RX LEDs (14): the board has two levels: 1) TX (transmit) and 2) RX (receive).

I/0 (15): the Arduino UNO board has 14 digital input/output pins, with six of them providing PWM output [5]. These digital pins have the ability to read logic values (0 and 1). A digital pin can power an L, E or D relay, for example.

AREF (16): the acronym AREF stands for analogue reference. It has a range of zero to five volts (Figure 10.9).

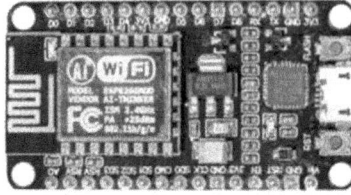

FIGURE 10.9   NodeMCU.

- The NodeMCU (node microcontroller unit) is an open source for development (hardware, software) platforms based on the ESP8266, a low-cost system-on-a-chip (SoC).

10.4.3.1   Advantages

1. Interactive
2. Programmable
3. Low cost
2. Simple interface
5. Smart IOT enabled with inbuilt Wi-Fi
6. Arduino compatible

10.4.3.2   Specifications

- Microcontroller: ESP-8266 32-bit
- NodeMCU model: Amica
- NodeMCU size: 49 mm x 26 mm
- Pin spacing: 0.9" (22.86 mm)
- Clock speed: 80 MHz
- USB to serial: CP2102
- USB connector: micro USB
- Operating: 3.3 V

Voltage:
- Input Voltage: 4.5 V–10 V
- Flash

Memory/SRAM: 4 MB/64 KB:
- Digital I/O pins: 11
- Analog pins: 1
- Wi-Fi built-in: 802.11 b/g/n

Power pins: There are four power pins—VINpin and three 3.3V pins.
- The NodeMCU/ESP8266 and its peripherals can be driven directly from VIN [6]. We can also use 5V controlled power can be supplied to the VIN pin (Figure 10.10) [7].

GND are the ground pins of NodeMCU/ESP8266.

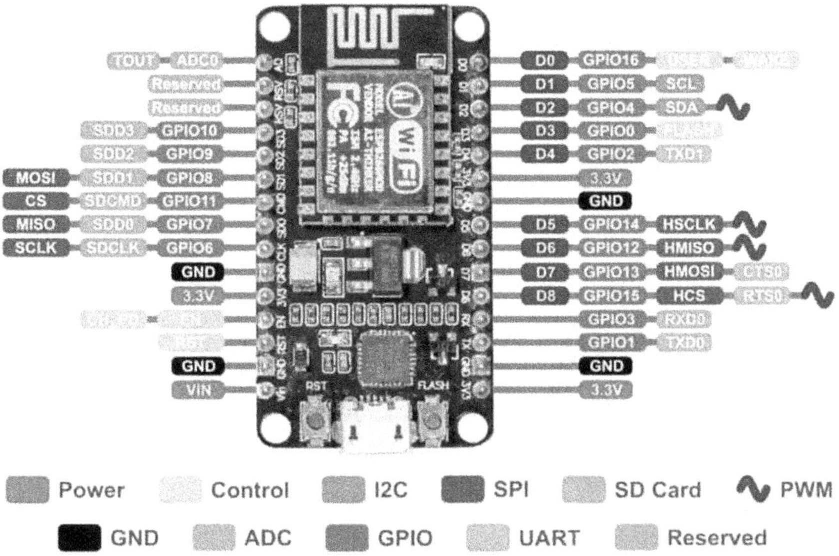

FIGURE 10.10   PIN diagram.

I2C pins: The I2C master and I2C slave functions are also supported [8].

GPIO pins: The 17 GPIO pins on the NodeMCU/ESP8266 can be programmatically assigned to functions

ADC Channel: 10-bit precision SAR ADC is built into the NodeMCU. ADC can be used to incorporate both functions. The VDD3P3 pin's power supply voltage is checked, as is the TOUT pin's input voltage. They cannot, however, be introduced at the same time.

UART pins: the NodeMCU/ESP8266 has two UART interfaces (UART0 and UART1) that support asynchronous (RS232 and RS485) communication at up to 4.5 Mbps [9].

SPI pins: NodeMCU/ESP8266 features two SPIs (SPI and HSPI) in slave and master modes. These SPIs also support the following general-purpose SPI features:

SDIO pins: NodeMCU/ESP8266 features a secure digital input/output interface (SDIO) which is used to directly interface SD cards.

PWM pins: the board has four channels of pulse width modulation (PWM) [10].

Control pins are used to control the NodeMCU/ESP8266. These pins include the chip enable pin (EN), reset pin (RST) and the WAKE pin.

- **EN**: the ESP8266 chip is on when EN pin is pulled to HIGH. When it is pulled to LOW the chip works at minimum power.
- **RST**: the RST pin is used to reset the ESP8266 chip [11].
- **WAKE**: the WAKE pin is used to wake the chip from deep sleep.
  - Control pins are used to control the NodeMCU/ESP8266.

10.4.4　L293 D Motor Driver

Motor drivers are devices that are used to control the motors in the automatic system. They are basically a bridge connecting the motors with the microcontroller. As the motor driver IC gets input from the controller in that way it drives the motors joined with it [12].

Very often used is the L293D model (Figures 10.11 and 10.12).

- ENABLE(1,2): used to enable input pins 1 and 2
- Input 1: controls the output 1
- Input 2: controls the output 2
- Output 1: connected to one end of motor 1
- Output 2: connected to another end of the motor 1
- Vec 2(V): this is relayed to the voltage pin of the running motors
- ENABLE(3,4): used to enable the input pins 3 and 4
- Input 3: controls the output 3
- Input 4: controls the output 4
- Output 3: connected to one end of motor 2
- Output 4: connected to another end of motor 2
- Vcc1(V): relayed to +5V

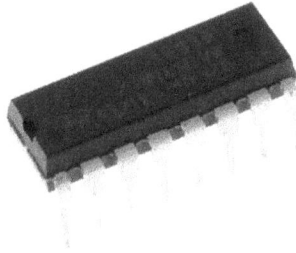

FIGURE 10.11　Motor driver.

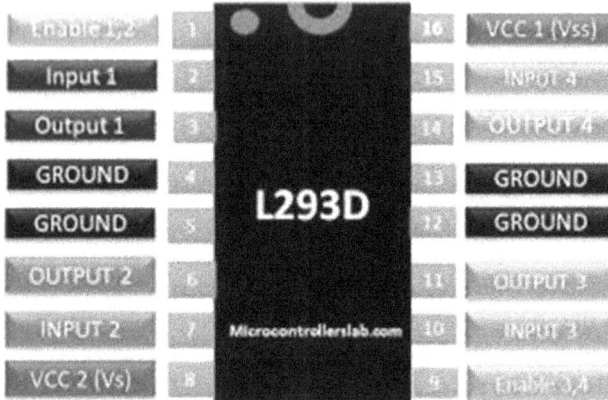

FIGURE 10.12　PIN configuration.

10.4.4.1 Features

- Two motors can run on a single IC board
- Speed and direction control can be attained
- Maximum voltage range: 4.5 V–36 V
- Maximum current (peak): 1.2 A
- Maximum continuous motor current: 600 Ma
- Supply voltage to Voc1 Vs: 4.5 v–7.0 v
- Transition time: 300 ns (at 5 V)

This driver can drive two motors simultaneously, and also, the direction control of the motors can be achieved through this driver [13].

The working principle of the driver is the half H bridge, which makes the movement of motors possible in both clockwise and anti-clockwise directions.

10.4.4.2 Applications of L293D

- This driver can be used in driving motors with high currents [14].
- Stepper motors too can be driven by these.

10.4.5 IR Sensors

Other application areas that use infrared sensors include (Figure 10.13):

- Climatology
- Meteorology
- Photobiomodulation
- Flame monitors
- Gas detectors
- Water analysis
- Moisture analysers
- Anesthesiology testing
- Petroleum exploration
- Rail safety
- Gas analysers

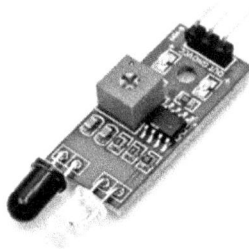

FIGURE 10.13 IR sensors.

10.4.6 TEMPERATURE SENSOR

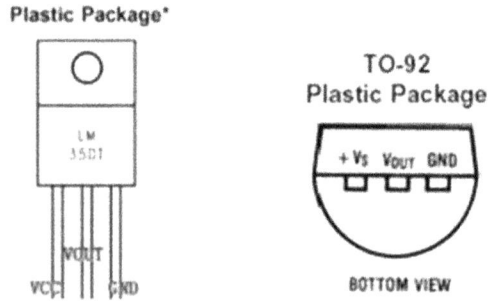

FIGURE 10.14 Temperature sensor.

10.4.6.1 Pin Configuration
- LM35 is a three-pin sensor
- The first pin is grounded
- The second pin is Vout
- The third pin is Vcc supply voltage
- Its input voltage is +5v in typical situations
- When it comes to output there will be an increase [15] of 10 millivolts for the raise of every 1 degree Celsius

10.4.6.2 Applications
- It can be used to measure the battery temperature
- It provides the battery protection from overheating
- It can be used in HVAC applications

10.4.6.3 Pin Configuration
- It is a three-pin sensor
- +3.3v = vcc
- Signal = output
- GND

10.4.6.4 Specification
- When the finger is on the sensor, the output response is pulse width modulation (Figure 10.15)
- When the finger is off to the sensor, the output response is a linear signal
- Operating voltage = +3.3v DC
- Operating current = 100 mA
- Output data level = 5v TTL
- Detection = indicated by LED and output high pulse
- Light source = 600 nm super red led

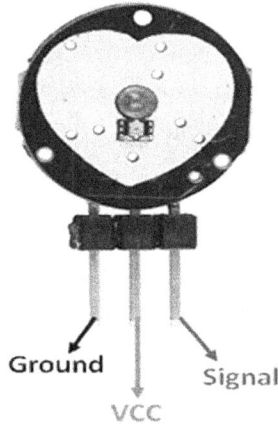

FIGURE 10.15 Heartbeat sensor.

10.4.6.5 Applications

- It is used in digital heart rate monitor systems like smartwatches and patient monitoring systems.
- It is used in biofeedback control of robotics and applications.

10.4.7 CALIBRATION OF TEMPERATURE SENSOR

It works under between −55 to +150 degrees Celcius.

$$V \propto T$$

V = 10mv
Below 0 degrees Celcius it is −ve voltage.
Temp c = V*0.1
Above 0 to 100 degrees Celcius
(Temp c*1.8) + 32
Vo = 2^10 = 1,024
ADC range from 0 to 10 v at maximum temperature is 100 degrees Celcius.

$$Vdd = +5v$$

Reference voltage with the connecting diode is = 1.2v.
Vo across the two diodes is = 1.196v
Surrounding temperature = 26.4 deg/c
Sensor Vo = 264 mv (0.264 v)

$$resolution = \frac{Vo\,cross\,diode}{Vo}$$

$$= \frac{1.196}{1024} = 0.00116$$

$$t = Vin \times resolution/V$$

$$= 226 \times 0.00168/(0.01) = 226 \times 0.168$$

$$= 37.9\,deg/c.$$

10.5　WORKING PRINCIPLE

- The working principle of the pick-and-place [16] robot depends on the wheels which are situated at the downside of the base part.
- Those wheels will help the robot to move in the desired path and location.
- Arduino UNO is the microcontroller for the pick-and-place robot, where all the components in the robot are controlled by the Arduino.
- There are two L293 D motor drivers in this robot; each motor driver can be responsible to drive the two DC motors.
- One motor driver will help to control the two DC motors in the pick-and-place robotic arm and another motor driver will help to drive the two motors which are connected to the two wheels.
- The wireless pick-and-place robot can be controlled in two ways: one is with the controller and another one is manually using the sensor.
- To control the robot manually, the Bluetooth module will be helpful. Where the Bluetooth module is connected to the microcontroller when we give the inputs [17] to the robot, it gets the signal from the controller to the Bluetooth module by taking the inputs we give and it assists the robot to give the output.
- The IR sensor detects the black line where the robot can move automatically by detecting the black line by emitting the heat.
- By thinking laterally, we got to know that according to several studies from Google we can use this kind of robotic application in hospitals near patients to bring necessary things or any kind of medical box.
- We can also make several updates to the robot in which it can be a patient-friendly robot.
- By fixing the two more sensors to the controller we can get the patients' basic data about their heartbeat and temperature.
- With the heartbeat sensor and the temperature sensor (LM35) of the Arduino UNO, we can check the patients' pulse rate and temperature.
- Where these two sensors are fixed to the robotic arm, when the patient places a hand on the sensor it will detect the input from the patient and give the output reading in the web application called ThingSpeak.
- In ThingSpeak, we are able to monitor the patient's health [18] condition from any place by signing in to ThingSpeak.
- To get the output readings in the ThingSpeak web application, the NodeMCU (Wi-Fi) module will help in this process.

10.5.1 Prototype Model

This model provides the overview of the actual working concept of the model. Figure 10.16 shows the prototype model of our work.

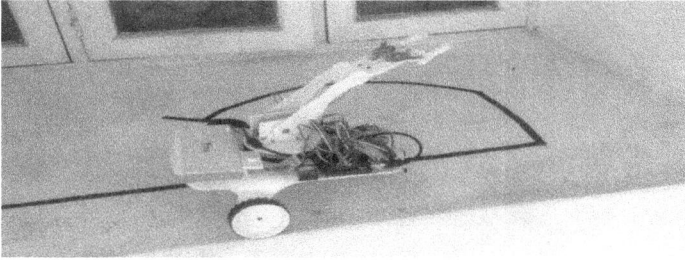

FIGURE 10.16 Prototype model.

10.5.2 Flow Charts

A flow chart provides the step, how the system works as shown in Figure 10.17.

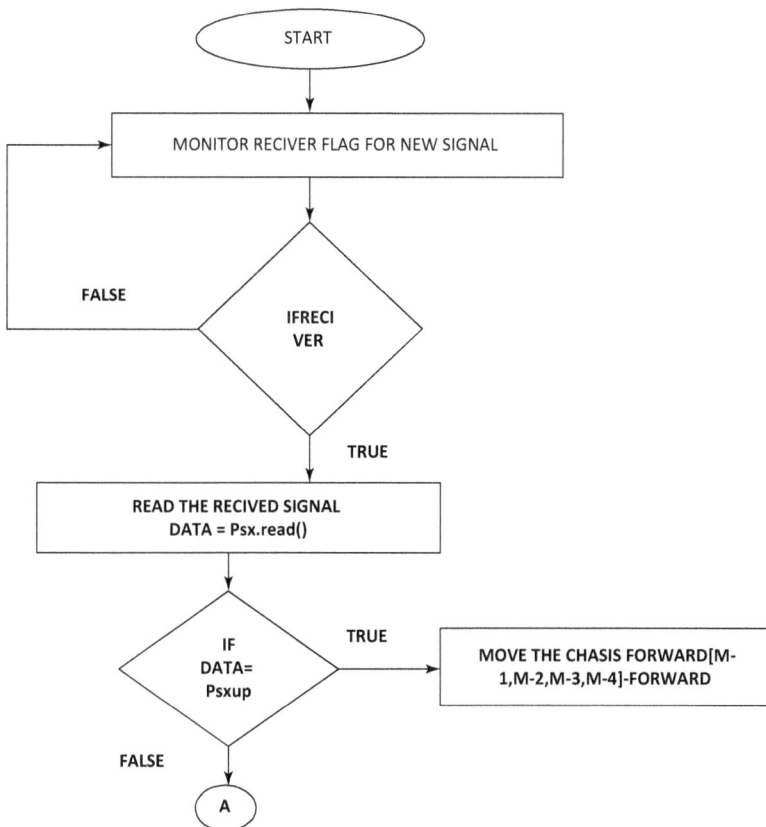

FIGURE 10.17 Data for receiving signal.

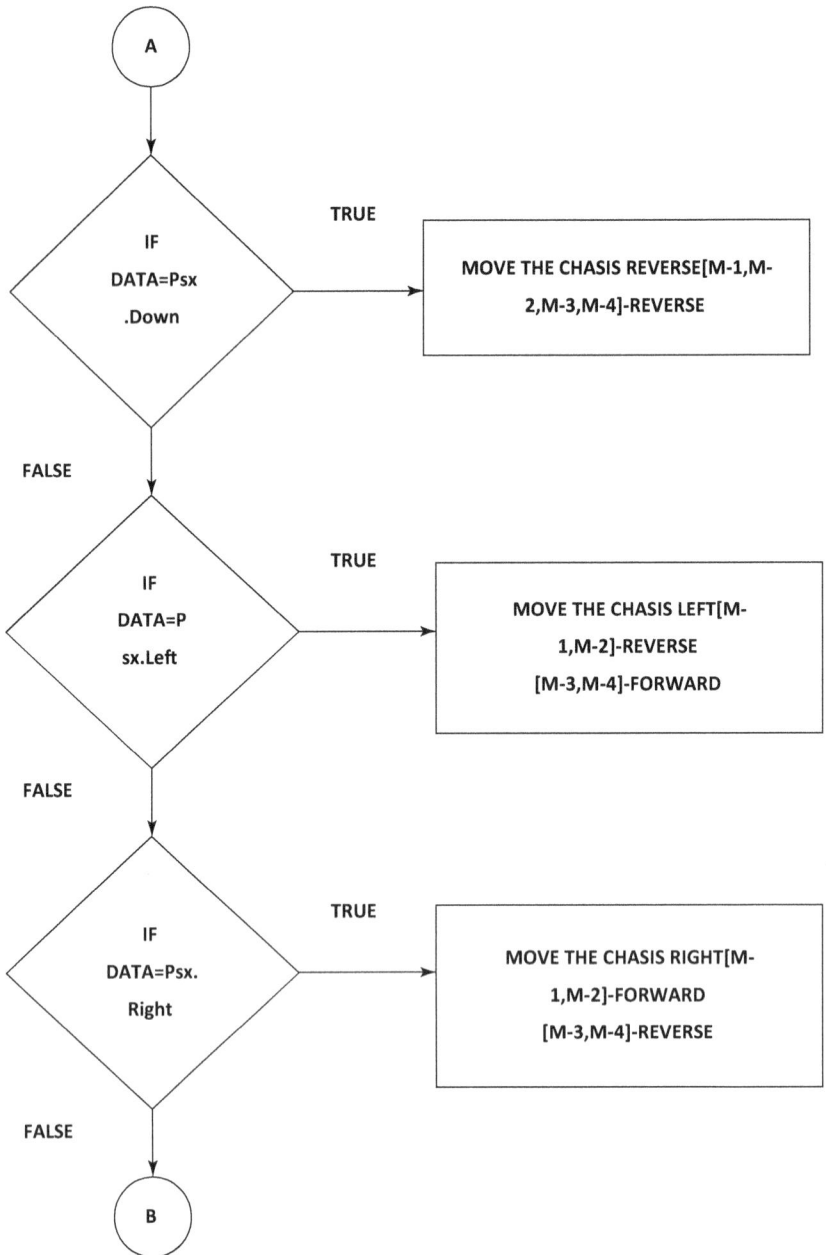

FIGURE 10.18   Diagram for defining process.

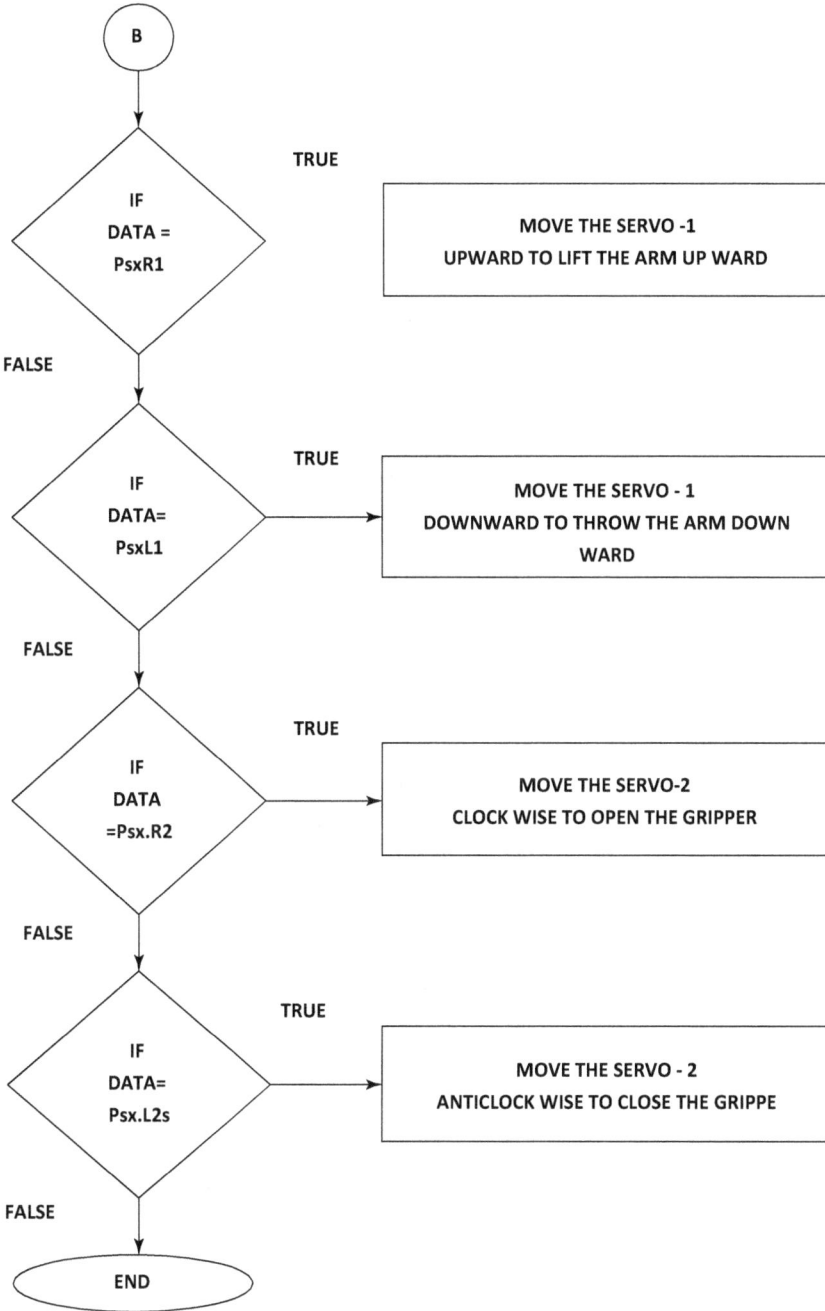

FIGURE 10.19   Diagram for defining flow of data.

10.6   CONCLUSION

The proposed pick-and-place robot idea utilising Arduino is intended for bedridden and older individuals. It is perceived that the robot has been presented and that it is equipped for moving itself to the position where the item to be raised is found, utilising a frame and four DC engines. It additionally lifts and positions the item depending on the controlling activity given to the servo engine.

10.7   FUTURE SCOPE

- This type of application can be used in hospitals near bedridden patients and in homes.
- It will be helpful for the bedridden people who want to lead an independent life.
- By keeping this kind of robotic application in hospitals, we can decrease the number of employees who monitor the patients for service.
- It is less in cost and has no power consumption.
- This robotic arm can also be used in surgery.
- In future, this kind of application will have a great life; in China some of the hospitals are using this kind of robotic application to serve the medicines for COVID-19 patients.

REFERENCES

1. S. Latif, J. Qadir, S. Farooq, and M. Imran, "How 5G wireless (and concomitant technologies) will revolutionize healthcare?" *Future Internet*, vol. 9, no. 4, p. 93, 2017.
2. Z. Yan, Y. Zhan, Z. Peng, S. Liao, Y. Shinagawa, S. Zhang, D. N. Metaxas, and X. S. Zhou, "Multi-instance deep learning: Discover discriminative local anatomies for body part recognition," *IEEE Transactions on Medical Imaging*, vol. 35, no. 5, pp. 1332–1343, 2016.
3. A. Kumar, D. Hung, D. Le, and T. Sairam, "Smart cities management using deep learning and IOT with cloud computing," *Global Journal on Innovation, Opportunities, and Challenges in Applied Artificial Intelligence and Machine Learning*, vol. 3, no. 1, 2019.
4. W. Książek, M. Abdar, U. Rajendra Acharya, and P. Pławiak, "A novel machine learning approach for early detection of hepatocellular carcinoma patients," *Cognitive Systems Research*, vol. 54, pp. 116–127, 2019.
5. B. Bratić, V. Kurbalija, M. Ivanović, et al., "Machine learning for predicting cognitive diseases: Methods, data sources, and risk factors," *Journal of Medical Systems*, vol. 42, p.243, 2018.
6. A. Kumar, S. Sharma, and S. Rasheed, "A shape mechanism along text-based advanced face detection methodology using EFM model," *IJIRCCE*, vol. 7, no. 2, p. 23209798, 2019.
7. J. Chaki, S. Thillai Ganesh, S. K. Cidham, et al., "Machine learning and artificial intelligence-based diabetes mellitus detection and self-management: A systematic review," *Journal of King Saud University – Computer and Information Sciences*.
8. U. Raghavendra, "Artificial intelligence techniques for automated diagnosis of neurological disorders,"

9. A. Dubey, S. Narang, A. Kumar, S. Sasubilli, and V. Díaz, "Performance estimation of machine learning algorithms in the factor analysis of COVID-19 dataset," *Computers, Materials & Continua*, 2020.

10. A. Segato, A. Marzullo, F. Calimeri, E. De Momi, "Artificial intelligence for brain diseases: A systematic review," *APL Bioeng*, vol. 4, no. 4, p. 041503, 2020. Published 2020 Oct 13. doi:10.1063/5.0011697.

11. Masud, M., Alhumyani, H., Alshamrani, S. S., Cheikhrouhou, O., Ibrahim, S., Muhammad, G., Shamim Hossain, M., and Shorfuzzaman, M., "Leveraging deep learning techniques for malaria parasite detection using mobile application", *Wireless Communications and Mobile Computing*, vol. 2020, Article ID 8895429, 15 pages, 2020. https://doi.org/10.1155/2020/8895429

12. N. Bhargava, A. K. Sharma, A. Kumar, and P. S. Rathoe, "An adaptive method for edge preserving denoising," in *2017 2nd International Conference on Communication and Electronics Systems (ICCES)*, Coimbatore, pp. 600–604, 2017. doi: 10.1109/CESYS.2017.8321149.

13. N. Bhargava, S. Sharma, R. Purohit, and P. S. Rathore, "Prediction of recurrence cancer using J48 algorithm," in *2017 2nd International Conference on Communication and Electronics Systems (ICCES)*, Coimbatore, pp. 386–390, 2017. doi: 10.1109/CESYS.2017.8321306.

14. Md. Sakibur Rahman Sajal, Md. Tanvir Ehsan, Ravi Vaidyanathan, Shouyan Wang, Tipu Aziz, and Khondaker Abdullah Al Mamun, "Telemonitoring Parkinson's Disease Using Machine Learning by Combining Tremor and Voice Analysis", *Brain Informatics*, vol. 7, no. 12, 2020, pp. 1–11. doi: 10.1186/s40708-020-00113-1.

15. C. K. Roopa, "A survey on various machine learning approaches for ECG analysis,"

16. M. Alloghani, A. Aljaaf, A. Hussain, T. Baker, J. Mustafina, D. Al-Jumeily, and M. Khalaf, "Implementation of machine learning algorithms to create diabetic patient re-admission profiles," *BMC Medical Informatics and Decision Making*, vol. 19, no. (Suppl 9), pp. 253, 2019 Dec 12. doi: 10.1186/s12911-019-0990-x. Erratum in: BMC Med Inform Decis Mak. 2020 May 18;20(1):93. PMID: 31830980; PMCID: PMC6907102.

17. S. Chandrasekaran, and A. Kumar, "Implementing medical data processing with Ann with hybrid approach of implementation," *Journal of Advanced Research in Dynamical and Control Systems – JARDCS*, vol. 10, pp. 45–52, 2018.

18. R. Raturi, and A. Kumar, "An analytical approach for health data analysis and finding the correlations of attributes using decision tree and W-logistic modal process," *IJIRCCE*, vol. 7, no. 6, 2019.

11 Challenges of Medical Text and Image Processing

G. Aparna, M. Kezia Joseph, S. Vani,
R. Srivel and Palvadi Srinivas Kumar

CONTENTS

11.1 INTRODUCTION

Transmission of delicate computerised information over remote correspondence channels has made it necessary for quick and secure advanced correspondence organisations to accomplish the needs for security, trustworthiness and non-disavowal during the time spent trading data. Cryptography gives a plan to getting and validating the transmission of data over shaky remote channels. It empowers us to store touchy data or communicate it across uncertain organisations with the goal that unapproved people can't get to the significant and classified information [1, 2]. The need for secure trade of advanced information brought about huge amounts of various encryption calculations which are assessed for equipment acknowledgement based on structure, calculation time, throughput, speed of activity and region

DOI: 10.1201/9781003132110-11

prerequisites. There are mostly two sorts of cryptographic calculations: symmetric and deviated calculations. A symmetric framework like Data Encryption Standard (DES), Triple-DES and Advanced Encryption Standard (AES) utilises an indistinguishable key for the sender and collector; both to encode the message and unscramble the code text. Image security enhancement is an important process for the rapid growth in communications technology. Digital data is being used in many applications such as medical, industrial, or even military applications and also multimedia applications [3]. The digital data can be interrupted by non-recipients over unsecured networks. Consequently, it is a very critical process to hide the multimedia content for transmission.

A cryptographic method is utilised to ensure information security. Ordinarily, cryptography is tied in with making and breaking down conventions that turn away outsiders from unauthorised users. The algorithm chosen and the cryptographic method employed must ensure fulfilling the cryptosystem general requirements.

Data assumes an indispensable part in the current period of advanced innovation. It is of different structures. Beginning from the content, pictures, it alludes to sound and video too. Writing study uncovers the presence of information innovation (might be in various structures) in antiquated occasions. The regal individuals propagate messages in encoded structures so that the beneficiary can unravel the transmitted information. Presently, advanced communication process, there is a high priority for channel coding methods to discover the best one for explicit applications. This chapter presents the research work of such a methodology for picture-based applications. During the previous few years, portable/remote frameworks have become predominant methods for correspondence. Their benefits, in any case, come at the expense of critical extra intricacy in the plan of reasonable channel coding and wireless transmission frameworks [4–6].

The particular use of picture transmission over remote channels represents a difficult exploration issue and proper choice of the arrangement of the above-mentioned powerful tools which are channel codes for future mistake rectification along with error control schemes. Computerised watermarking is an effective instrument to forestall the unauthenticated utilisation of information. Advanced watermarks might be utilised to confirm the genuineness or trustworthiness of the first information. These days, it is unmistakably utilised for following copyright encroachments and for banknote verification. Computerised watermarking is comprehensively arranged to rely upon the kind of signs like sound watermarking, picture watermarking, video watermarking and information-based watermarking and so forth. The current work is centred around picture watermarking. In picture watermarking, the computerised data (like an advanced picture, an advanced signature or an arbitrary arrangement of parallel numbers) is installed into a picture. The implanted data might possibly be noticeable subsequent to watermarking and in this manner falls into the classification of apparent or imperceptible watermarking separately. Contingent upon the strength of the watermark, it can likewise be classified as hearty or delicate watermarking. One impediment of watermarking-based verification plans is the twisting caused on the host media by the implanting cycle. Albeit the twisting is frequently inconsequential, it may not be adequate for certain applications, particularly in the space of clinical imaging and military applications. Consequently, the watermarking plan is fit for eliminating the contortion and recuperating.

With fast expansion in the use of web and computerised media, transmission and propagation of advanced items have gotten advantageous; however, there are a few disadvantages too. The computerised unrest gives devices to limitless replicating without misfortune in constancy. Individuals can without much of a stretch take the computerised work of others like pictures, recordings and brief snippets and guarantee their privileges on the taken things.

Watermark (WM) has different structures, for example, content worth, picture, video and brief snippet. WM method has a few properties to be characterised like vigour, security, intricacy, check and so forth. Strength is a significant property since it characterises the endurance of the watermark in watermarked computerised media. The watermarking framework can be executed with one or the other programming or equipment. Programming execution of watermarking is enormous while equipment execution is deficient. For the most part, an equipment watermarking plan should be possible by utilising every one of the areas (spatial or recurrence). Because of the straightforwardness of spatial space computational overhead and its effectiveness for its application whenever contrasted with the recurrence area, the spatial space is generally liked for equipment execution. The expansion of digitised media (sound, picture and video) is making a squeezing need for copyright authorisation. Ordinary cryptographic frameworks grant just substantial key holders admittance to scrambled information, yet once such information is unscrambled, it is basically impossible to follow its propagation or retransmission. Subsequently, ordinary cryptography gives little security against information robbery, in which a distributor is stood up to with unapproved multiplication of data. A computerised watermark is planned to supplement cryptographic cycles.

It's anything but a noticeable, or ideally undetectable, recognisable proof code that is for all time inserted in the information and stays present inside the information after any decoding cycle. With regards to this work, information alludes to sound (discourse and music), pictures (photos and designs) and video (films). It does exclude ASCII portrayals of text, yet incorporates text addressed as a picture.

11.1.1 WATERMARKING

Advanced media can be replicated and changed effectively so securing the copyright of computerised media has become a significant undertaking. The computerised watermark is acquainted with taking care of the issue of copyright. Advanced watermarking is a strategy of inserting any watermark picture into a cover picture utilising some realised calculations relying on the necessity in sight and sound information to distinguish the proprietor of the document. There are two normal strategies for watermarking: spatial area and change space. In spatial space, pixels of a picture are adjusted, relying on perceptual examination of a picture. In any case, in the change area, a few frequencies are chosen and adjusted from their unique qualities as indicated by specific standards.

A summed up watermarking model comprises of two cycles: watermark implanting and recognition, as displayed in Figure 11.1.

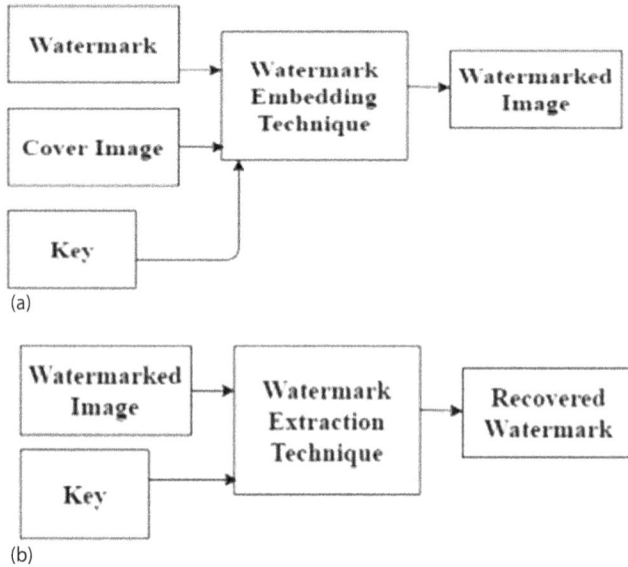

FIGURE 11.1   (a) Watermark embedding. (b) Watermark detection.

A watermark is an apparent or imperceptible mark installed inside a picture to show legitimacy or evidence of proprietorship. The secret watermark ought to be indistinguishable from the host picture, adequately vigorous to oppose any controls while protecting the picture quality. In this manner, through watermarking, scholarly properties stay available while being forever stamped. These computerised signature approaches used in verifying proprietorship assertions and securing restrictive secret data debilitate unapproved replicating and dissemination of pictures over the web and guarantee an advanced picture has not been changed. In this way, watermarking is primarily a concept of illegal duplicates or claims the responsibility for media. There are fundamental elements which make watermarking successful, mentioned below.

- *Vigour*: A watermark ought to be hard to eliminate or obliterate. It's essentially a proportion of invulnerability of the watermark against endeavours of picture adjustment and control like pressure, sifting, revolution, impact assaults, resizing, trimming, and so on.
- *Indistinctness*: The nature of the host picture ought not to be annihilated by the presence of a watermark.
- *Limit*: It incorporates procedures that make it conceivable to insert a larger amount of data.

11.1.2   DIGITAL WATERMARKING EMBEDDING AND EXTRACTION PROCESS

In the inserting interaction, the watermark might be encoded into the cover picture utilising a particular key. This key is utilised to encode the watermark as an extra insurance level. The yield of the implanting interaction, the watermarked picture, is then communicated to the beneficiary. In the discovery interaction likewise called an extraction measure, the watermark is retrieved very near to the original one without getting corrupted. Figure 11.1a, b shows the block diagram of watermark embedding and watermark detection, respectively.

11.1.3　Turbo Encoder: Convolution Codes

In recent channel coding techniques evolution convolutional codes are well known for error correction capability that is achieving Shannon capacity. The idea of these codes works with lattice disentangling utilising a period invariant lattice. This is as opposed to exemplary square codes, which are for the most part addressed by a period variation lattice and hence are commonly hard-choice decoded. Convolutional codes are frequently described by the base code rate and the profundity (or memory) of the encoder (n, k, K).

Convolutional codes are somewhat similar to the square codes talked about in the past address in that they include the transmission of equality bits that are processed from message bits. Not at all like square codes in efficient structure, notwithstanding, the sender doesn't send the message bits followed by (or sprinkled with) the equality bits; in a convolutional code, the sender sends just the equality bits. The encoder utilises a sliding window to figure r > 1 equality bits by joining different subsets of pieces in the window. The joining is a basic expansion in F2, as in the past addresses (i.e. modulo 2 expansion, or proportionately, a selective or activity). Not at all like a square code, the windows cover and slide by 1, as displayed in Figure 11.8. The size of the window, in bits, is known as the code's limitation length. The more extended the requirement length, the bigger the number of equality bits that are impacted by some random message bit. Since the equality pieces are the lone pieces sent over the channel, a bigger limitation length, by and large, suggests a more prominent strength to bit mistakes. The compromise, however, is that it will take significantly more to interpret codes of long limitation length, so one can't build the requirement length subjectively and anticipate quick deciphering.

The fundamental reason for the interleaver is to build the base distance of the turbo code with the end goal that after amendment in one measurement the excess mistakes should become correctable blunder designs in the subsequent measurement. Disregarding for the moment the deferral for each square, we accept both encoders yield information all the while. This is rate 1/3 turbo code, the yield of the turbo encoder being the trio (Xk, Y1k and Y2k).

The essential thought of super codes is to utilise two convolutional codes in corresponding with some sort of interleaving in the middle. Convolutional codes can be utilised to encode a constant stream of information, yet for this situation, we accept that information is designed in limited squares—relating to the interleaver size. The edges can be ended—for example, the encoders are compelled to a known state after the data block. The end tail is then added to the encoded data and utilised in the decoder. The framework is represented in Figure 11.2.

It can be observed that the super code is a huge square code. The exhibition relies upon the weight conveyance—the base distance as well as the number of words with

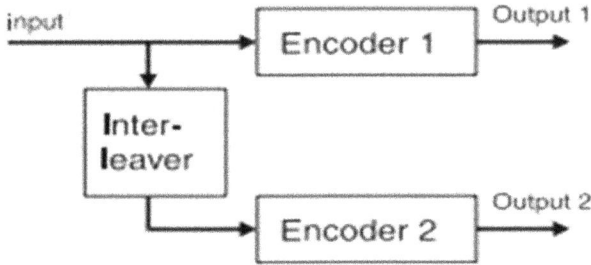

FIGURE 11.2 Turbo encoder.

low weight. The turbo encoder gives a yield of 28 pieces which is a blend of information and a yield of two RSC encoders which is threefold the length of the information bits as is displayed in Figure 11.3.

11.1.4 INTERLEAVER

The interleaver plan is a major block involved in error-correcting factors, which decides the demonstration of a turbo code. Shannon showed that enormous square length irregular codes accomplish channel limits. When contrasted with the other interleaver, it is straightforward and simple to implement. A square interleaver composes information in a grid line from left to right and through and through. After all the data pieces are composed into a lattice, it peruses the information in segments. The output of the interleaver is given to RSC2 as shown in Figure 11.3.

Recent trends in digital image processing approaches over wireless channels globally have increased various demands of providing security for the data communications for transmission and reception of information for medical applications, which is drawing the attention of researchers in security, implementation and algorithmic selection points of view [7, 8]. Technology development in medical applications requires knowledge of advances in computing and computer-based communication for providing health services. Telemedicine is a modern way of medical healthcare for Internet of Things–driven healthcare applications that can be extended to any remote place across the globe [9].

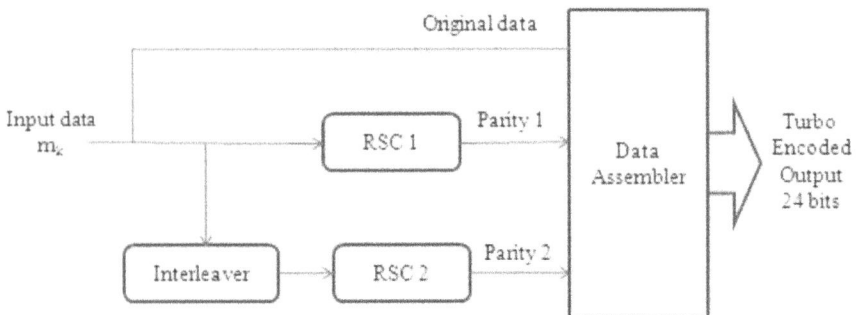

FIGURE 11.3 Turbo encoder block diagram.

However, this exchange of information is confined by several risks of data theft when the data are shared in open networks and hence they are to be protected with high-security algorithms. This chapter provides a high-capacitive security algorithm for protecting medical images with hidden clinical information.

In the process of medical image transmission, the following are the challenges with the experimental investigations, presented with the prior work done and discussed in the section below.

11.2 LITERATURE SURVEY

11.2.1 STATEMENT OF THE PROBLEM AND OVERCOMING SECURITY PROBLEMS

The main challenge is to propose a model for robust transmission of medical text over wireless channels with security in a reliable and authenticated mode. For providing robustness, channel coding techniques can be used and for reliability and authentication encryption techniques can be employed. These would enhance the security as well as assure authentication also. In this chapter, a thorough review of encryption techniques like the Advanced Encryption Standard (AES) algorithm, a well-known and widely used block cypher for emerging cryptographic applications in information security scenarios. An efficient AES algorithm is designed and developed for patient raw data. The first step in this thesis is encryption of the patient raw data with a 128-bit AES algorithm [10–12]. The user key can't be directly taken as input for the encryption process. A key generation block is included to generate whole ten-round keys for encryption. With this rapid enhancement, hackers can't decrypt the data even though the original key of the encrypted algorithm is known.

11.2.2 PROVIDING STRENGTHENING TO ENCRYPTION

Through the encryption process, data is converted into an unreadable format. With that cypher text, the admin reveals to hackers that space transmission data is encrypted by using secured algorithms [13, 14] so that hackers can try to decrypt the data with all his/her aspects. In order to avoid hackers' trails, we need some sophisticated system to keep the data as it is in some other original information. Invisible watermarking plays a significant role in that scenario. So, watermarking with a cover image using the discrete wavelet transform technique is used for providing more strengthening to AES-encrypted data [15–17].

11.3 CHALLENGE 1: RELIABLE COMMUNICATION

Nowadays, all communications are very high speed, powerful and wireless. So, channels are not that robust and reliable. Error occurrence probability increases in day-to-day life with an increase in different faults types. Efficient channel encoders and decoders are needed in order to rectify or correct those errors. Turbo encoders are very much efficient in solving these types of errors especially in communication errors [18–22]. The cryptosystem for reliable communication also includes key establishment, trust issues and authentication too. In the prior proposed technique

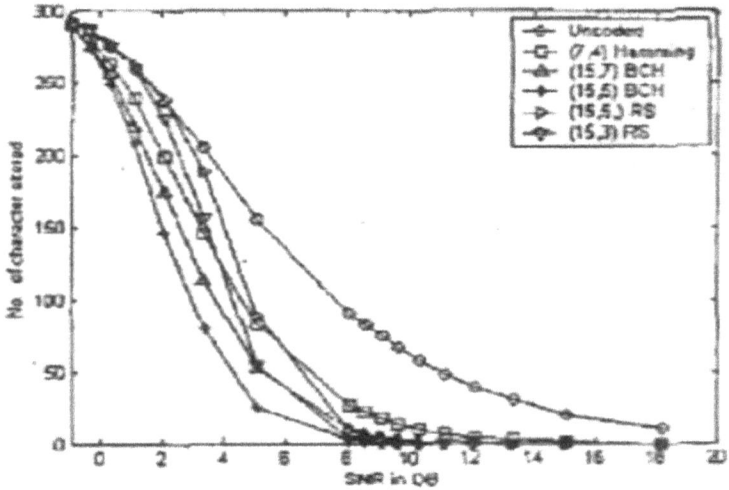

FIGURE 11.4 Graph representing the NOCA in the literature.

for dependable and robust transmission [23, 24] strategy, the hysterical situation is recreated by adding salt and pepper commotion to the implanted picture for various SNR of the picture, BER and NOCA for text information and rate twisting for the sign chart. The coded frameworks can perform better compared to the encoded frameworks. Figure 11.4 represents the NOCA graphically.

   This is the inspiration for picking ECC to communicate the information, particularly clinical data of the patient which has crucial information.

11.3.1 CHALLENGE 2: SECURED COMMUNICATION

The latest encryption algorithm, Rijndael, is used for encrypting text information. Signal graphs like ECG, EEG and EMG were used for compression techniques.

   G. Aparna et al. have proposed a secured approach for processing the ECG signals in which the signal is acquired and decomposed using DWT to obtain approximated and detailed coefficients [25, 26]. The approximated terms are compressed and the detailed coefficients are encrypted using the RSA algorithm and transmitted so as to store in the data repository for a patient-centric approach. This method has shown that the compression ratio achieved is 2.71.

   Later, the work for machine learning concepts was extended where the PSNR and MSE values were evaluated for the performance measure of the image processing over wireless channels for analysis.

11.3.2 CHALLENGE 3: ROBUST TRANSMISSION

To enhance the robustness of the embedded information, the patient information is coded by error-correcting codes [27, 28]. Here in the proposed approach, turbo codes are used for error control.

11.3.2.1 Objective

The information to be stored is encrypted before watermarking [29–34] to enhance security. AES is the well-known standard for the encryption of text data developed by the National Institute of Standards and Technology (NIST) (Figure 11.4).

Figure 11.5 denotes the various levels of the encryption process implemented on the medical image for the defined iterations.

Figure 11.6 represents the curve of the bit error rate with turbo coding and without turbo coding.

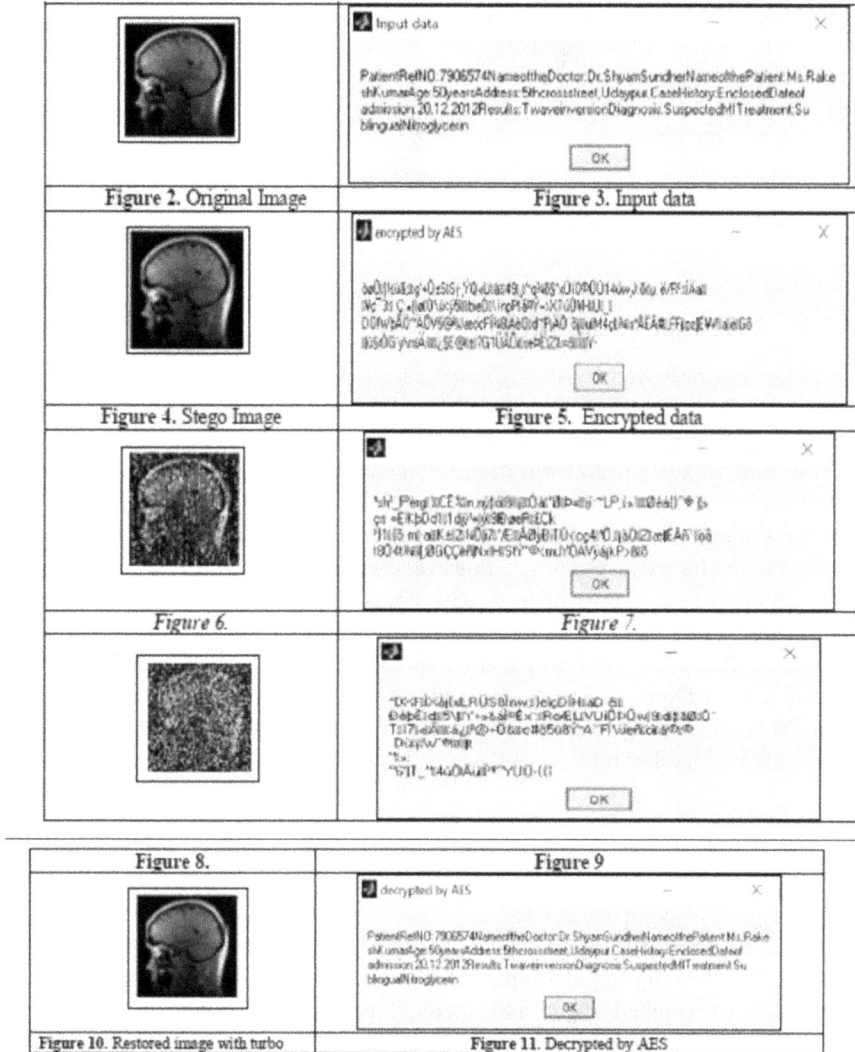

Figure 2. Original Image	Figure 3. Input data
Figure 4. Stego Image	Figure 5. Encrypted data
Figure 6.	Figure 7.
Figure 8.	Figure 9
Figure 10. Restored image with turbo	Figure 11. Decrypted by AES

FIGURE 11.5   AES encryption implementation on plain text for medical applications.

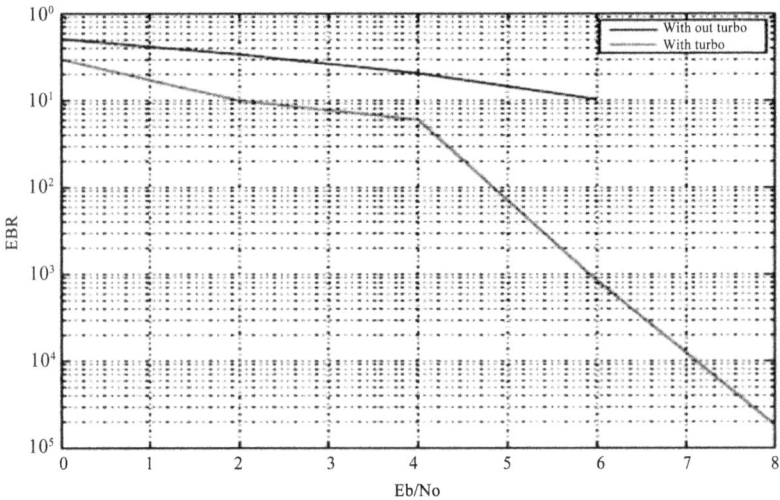

FIGURE 11.6 BER curve of the AES encryption with channel coding and without coding.

11.3.3 CHALLENGE 4: ALGORITHM

The algorithm provided by Prof Deergha Rao is able to embed a binary image within a medical image of size 32×24 and get the host image to be 128×128 or 256×256. The extraction algorithm is able to retrieve the details from the watermarked image and to form the embedded logo or image but the bit error is not zero.

Since the embedded image [35–38] is a binary image we could not find much difference in the extracted logo; however, when the bit error is calculated it shows an error rate of 0.01 or more. So this is not suitable when the embedded part is text.

A minor change in a bit may change the alphanumeric value, which is clearly depicted in the tst2.png image shown in Figure 11.7 and Figure 11.8, respectively.

So, therefore, the technique could be able to extract the same original data which is embedded with other images [39].

11.3.4 CHALLENGE 5: COMPACT STORAGE

In challenge 5 of compact storage, the vital information of the patient details is converted into ASCII form and stored. Figure 11.9 gives the pseudo-code written in MATLAB showing the text input reading process in the file form and encrypting the data, then embedding it in the medical image. The encrypted output and the watermarked image are shown in Figure 11.10 and the observation made from the outputs and the motivation of the work towards the proposed scheme of approach are shown.

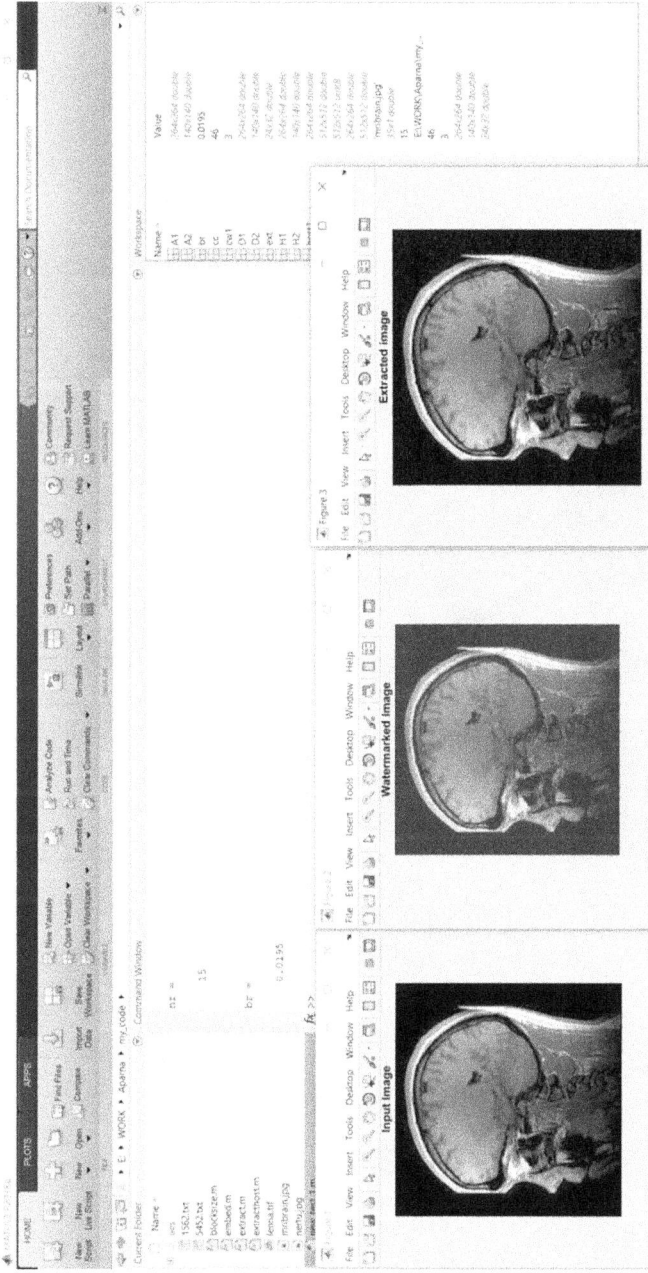

FIGURE 11.7 Experimental investigations of exisiting algorithm implementation indicating the challenges and scope.

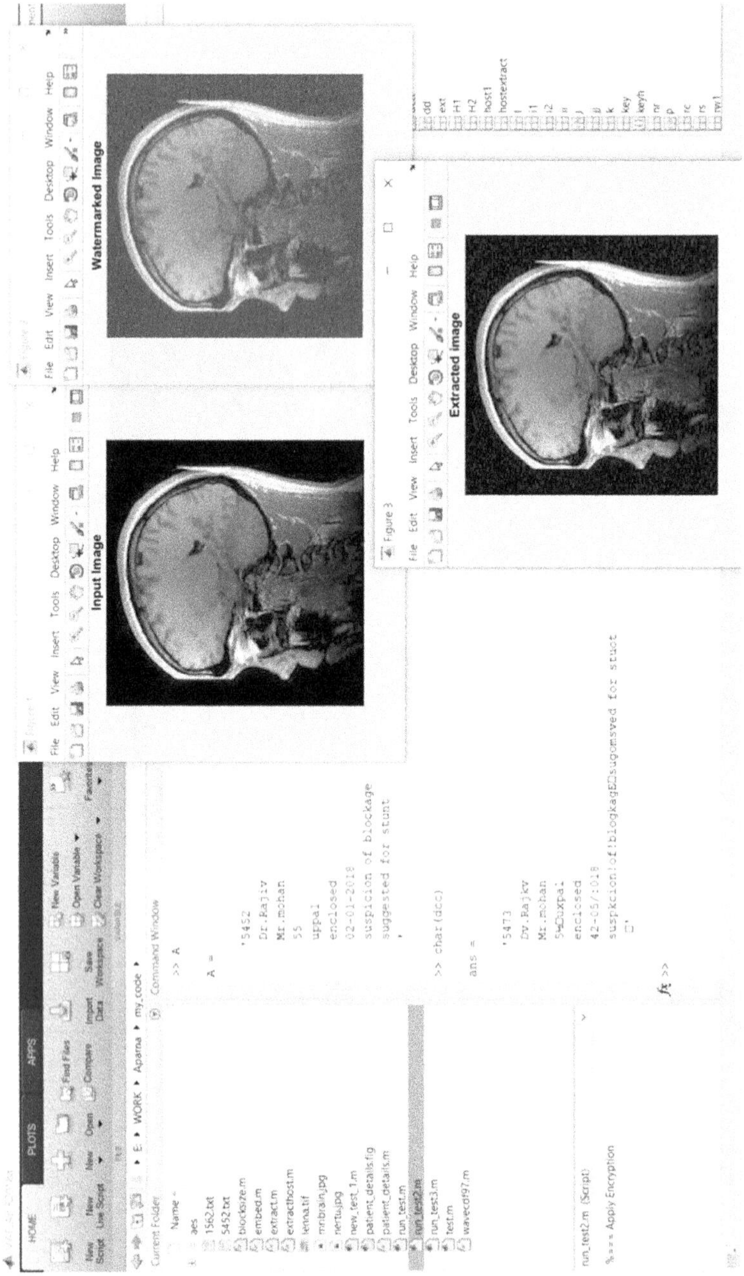

FIGURE 11.8   Test results and challenges observed in the implementation of existing related works.

```
clc
clear all
close all
% Reading the image
img = imread('mribrain.jpg');
img1 = zeros(size(img));
img1 = (double(img));
img2 = (double(img));
i=1;imshow(img)
y = [];
%reading a file
file=fopen('apar.txt','rb');
while ~feof(file)
    x=fscanf(file,'%c',1);
    y = [y x];
end
fclose(file);
ln = length(y);
y1 = double(uint8(y));
% encrypting the data
itc = ((log(10*2)*100)-300);
ye = char(uint8((log(y1*2)*100)-300));
img1(1:ln) = ((log(y1*2)*100)-300);
fid = fopen('newfile.txt','wb');
fprintf(fid, '%s', char(uint8(img1(1:ln))));
fclose(fid);
figure,imshow(uint8(img1))
yd = (img1(1:ln));%char
yd8 = double(uint8(yd));
ydd=exp((yd8+300)/100-log(2));%*ct
ydd = char(uint8(ydd));
 %decrypted data
 fid = fopen('newfile.txt','rb');
yd = [];
while ~feof(file)
    x=fscanf(file,'%c',1);
    yd = [yd x];
end
fclose(fid);
```

FIGURE 11.9 MATLAB coding to encrypt the plain text in image.

11.4 PROPOSED APPROACH FOR MEDICAL TEXT AND IMAGE PROCESSING

The approach is a hybrid security [40] technique for IoT healthcare applications that provides two-way security by encrypting the clinical information initially and embedding it imperceptibly in the concerned image so that the user on the other side can obtain both the visual and text data at the same instance. In the secret data communication system model, the encrypted and watermarked image is communicated over a wireless channel which may be corrupted due to noise. This initiates to encode the data with an error-correcting code so as to retain the image quality and hence better performance measurement parameters in terms of BER and PSNR. Figure 11.11 shows the GUI designed using MATLAB to enter the patient clinical information.

ye = 'ÐãöëçïõtÒçètíî‾tª®œ¨ªº Íãîçtðètõêçt¿ðåõõó‾t¿ó~ÓêùãîtóÖö ïæêçót ÍãîçtðètõêçtÐãöëçïõ‾tîô~ÒãíçôêtÉ öîãót »éç‾ œùçãóó »ææóçôô‾ öêtåóðõôtôõõóççõ"tÖææâ ùñöó~ ¾ãôçtÅëôõõóù‾tÁïãîôôçæ ¿ãõçtðètãæîëôôëõï‾ œ~ ¡~¡œ ¡ Òçööîõô‾Ôt÷ãöçtëïöçóôëõï ¿ëãéïõõëô‾tÓööñçåõçætÌÆ Óóçãõîçïõ‾tÓöäíëïéöãîtÍëõóóõéîùå çóëï'	
ydd = 'Patient Ref NO: 7906574 Name of the Doctor: Dr.Shyam Svndher Name of the Patient: Ms.Rakesh Kvmar Age:50years Address:5th cross street, Udaypvr. Case History: Encmosed Date of admission:20.12.2012 Resvmts:T wave inversion Diagnosis: Svspected MI Treatment: Svbmingvam Nitrogmycerin'	**Observation**: From the output figures and the results displayed on the command window while executing the above mentioned Matlab code it is observed that a few alphabets or characters got altered which is termed of NOCA (Number of Characters Altered) which is not at all permissiable for medical applications. This is the major challenge in medical text and image processing to send the data in a secured manner and to retrieve it without any distortion or loss of information. The access should be only for authorised persons and the retrieval must be error free. **Motivation:** Hence there is a high demand for error correction schemes and also the algorithm should be robust and must achieve appreciable performance measures in terms of PSNR and BER.

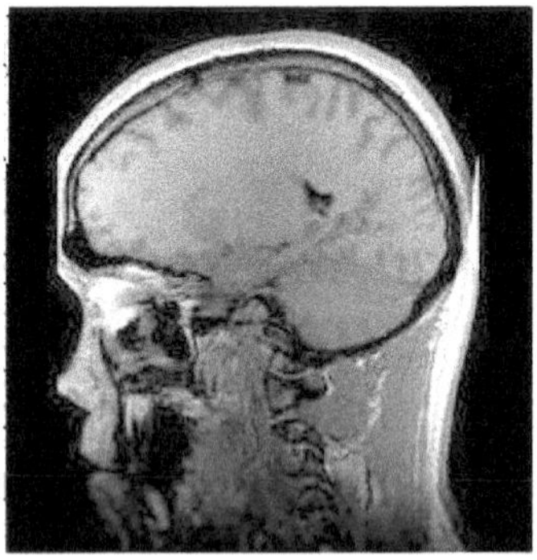

FIGURE 11.10   Executed outputs of the plain text and observations.

Figure 11.12 gives the original data and the encrypted data of the medical information of the patient which is taken is as input.

The experiments were conducted on different medical images like MR brain image, CT abdominal image and lung X-ray image. The proposed approach is compared against the method proposed by Elhoseny and others [41]. The results are shown in Figure 11.13, mentioning the PSNR values representing the performance metrics of the proposed approach for the images of X-ray, CT-scan and MRI input images. Figures 11.14–11.17 denote the BER curve, the PSNR curve and the comparative curve, respectively, for various input images and their performances with and without channels, namely turbo codes.

The decrypted information of the proposed method is shown in Figure 11.18 for the original information taken as input and the encrypted process of the information.

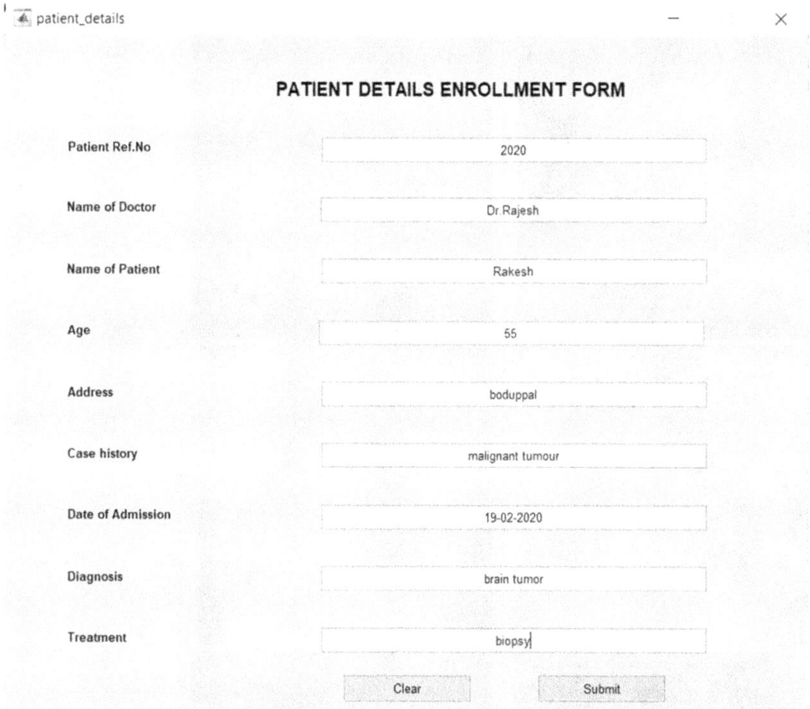

FIGURE 11.11 GUI to enter the patient text details in the entry form showing clinical information.

From the graph, it is to be observed the proposed mechanism yielded a high-quality stego image with high capacity. In Figure 11.2, different medical images when passed through an AWGN channel achieve very low BER; it is further reduced when turbo coding is incorporated with the model. The hiding capacity for the developed approach was justified against the method proposed by Elhoseny [41–44] who observed the proposed approach attains high-quality imperceptible images which are approximately 1.9 dB improved on average. This highlights the objective of the

Original Data	Encrypted Data
2020 Dr.Rajesh Rakesh 55 boduppal malignant tumour 19-02-2020 brain tumor biopsy	x »(æ!*œ¥ÉLöt¿#"ÊT^›Øñv¤éó ~¢zJÔ ⁻Ø—‚ã*T²†ôì»>Š9ëÂ8jŠÎV¿NôË]|è —& —+:&øí

FIGURE 11.12 Outputs of the original text and the encrypted outputs.

Image	Stego-Image	PSNR
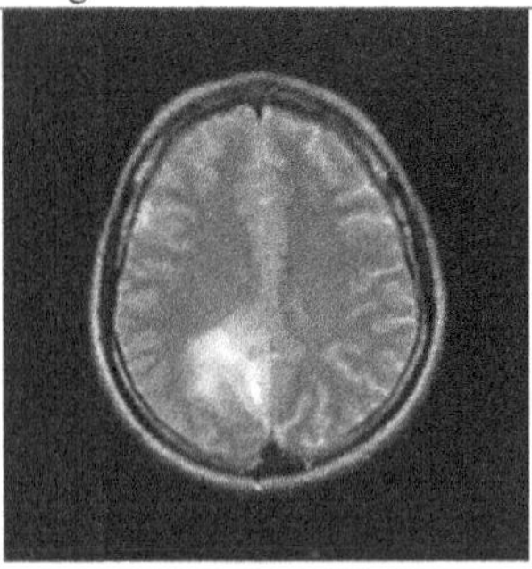	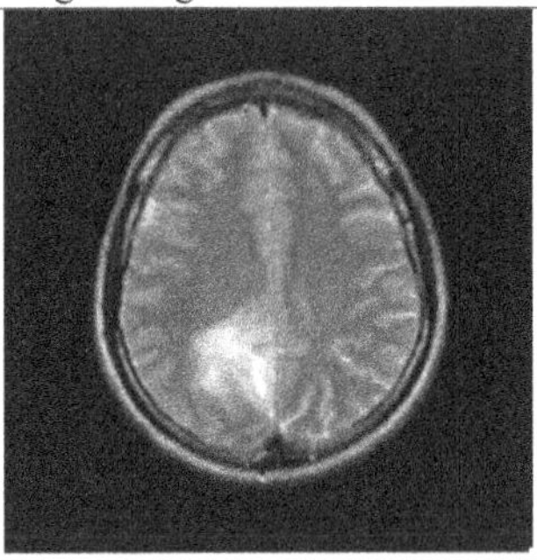	49.03
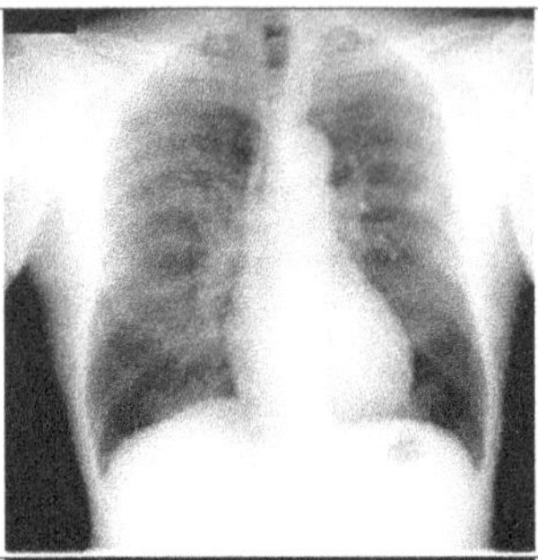	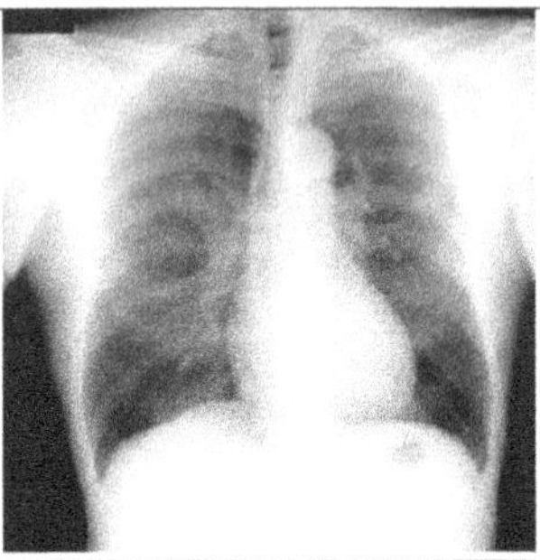	48.46
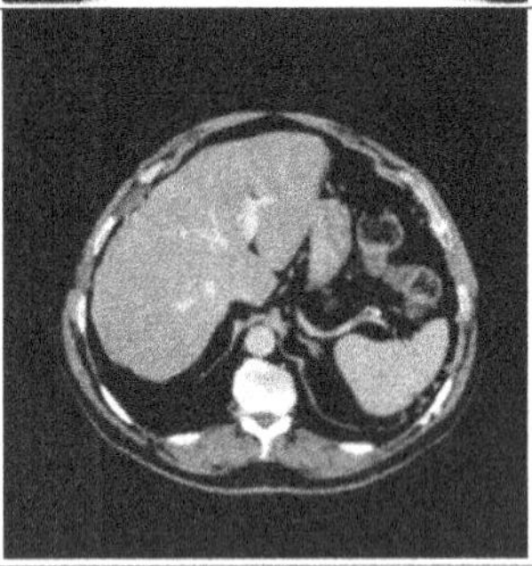	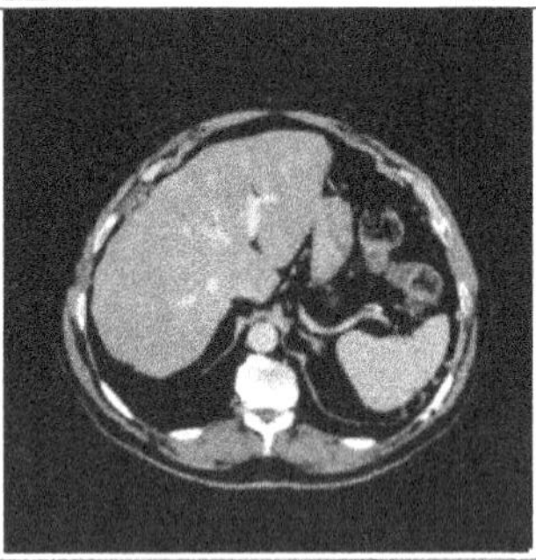	47.44

FIGURE 11.13   Performance metrics of the proposed approach.

current of achieving a high-capacity, secure and imperceptible medical image transmission model.

11.5   CONCLUSIONS

The chapter presents various problems in medical text- and image-processing mechanisms and also a method to handle the situation in a secured and high-capacity medical image transmission manner with a suggestible model that attains high-quality imperceptible stego-images which are transmitted through an AWGN channel. In this work, the BER analysis was considered with and without turbo coding and found that with the coding mechanism included, the BER is very low and suitable

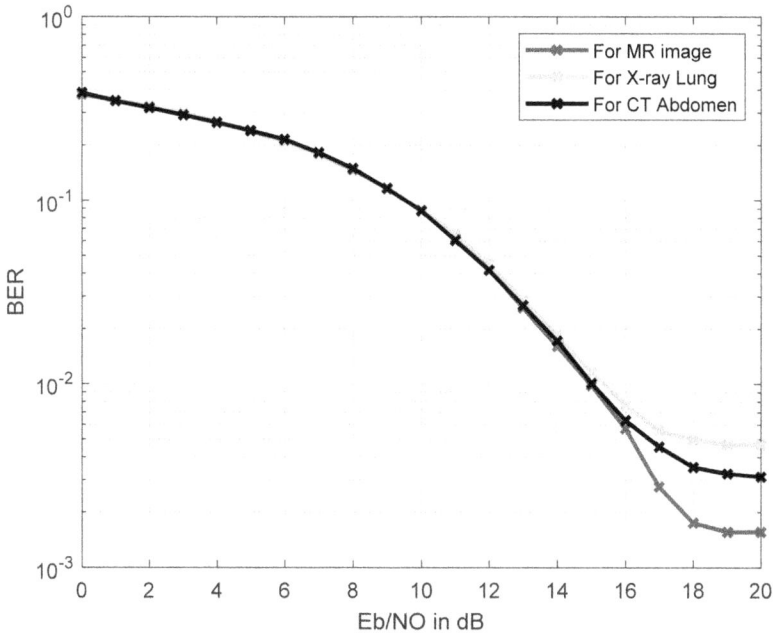

FIGURE 11.14 BER performance of multiple medical images with varying Eb/NO under AWGN channel.

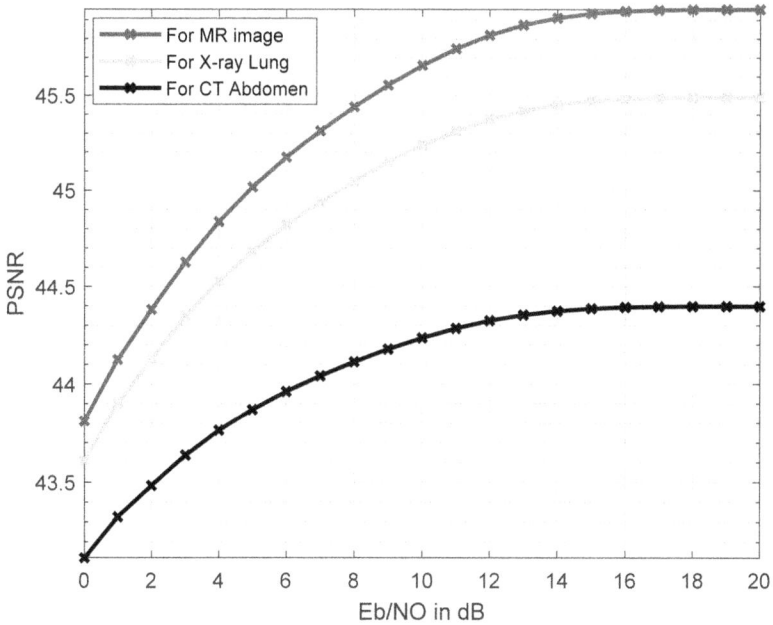

FIGURE 11.15 PSNR performance of multiple medical images with varying Eb/NO under AWGN channel.

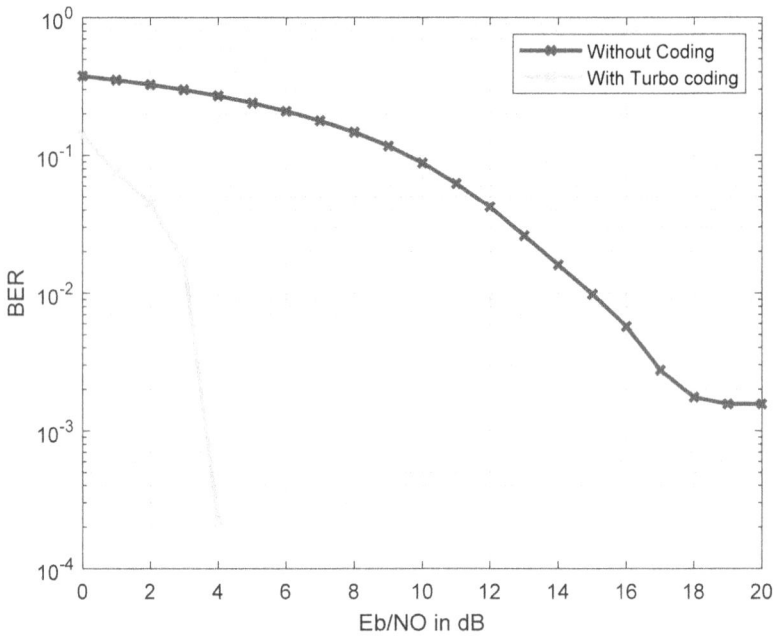

FIGURE 11.16 BER performance of MR medical image with varying Eb/NO under AWGN channel with and without turbo coding.

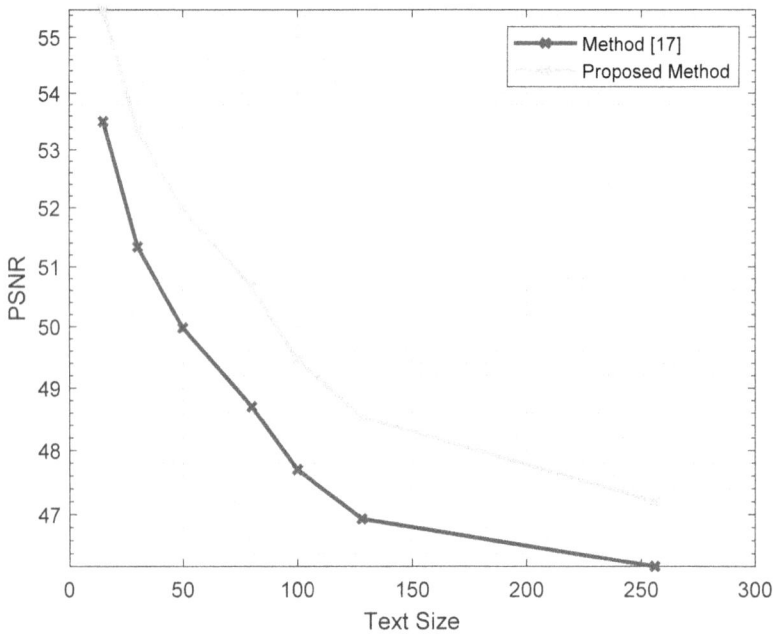

FIGURE 11.17 PSNR performance of MR medical image with varying text size and comparison with method proposed in [41].

Original Information	Encrypted Information	Decrypted Information
2020 Dr.Rajesh Rakesh 55 boduppal malignant tumour 19-02-2020 brain tumor biopsy	x »(æ!*œ¥ÉLöt¿#"ÊT^›Øñv¤éó ~¢zJÔ ¯Ø—¸ã*T²†ôì»>Š9ëÂ8jŠÎV¿NôË]|è —& –+:&øí	2020 Dr.Rajesh Rakesh 55 boduppal malignant tumour 19-02-2020 brain tumor biopsy

FIGURE 11.18   Clinical patient diagnostic details encryption and decryption output.

for real-time application. The work mainly tries to propose a high capacitive and imperceptible mode of medical image transmission which is achieved when compared with earlier methods. The hardware realisation [45–48] of the approach gives the hardware components required for the implementation of the proposed method to achieve the required speed, throughput and delay parameters for advanced signal processing applications in wireless communications. The scope of the challenges is extended to hardware implementation depicting the digital components required for the realisation of the proposed challenges of medical text and image processing. The simulation and synthesis results of the hardware approach are presented as the next upcoming challenge.

REFERENCES

1. C. E. Shannon, "A mathematical theory of communication," *The Bell System Technical Journal*, July 1948, 27, pp. 379–423.
2. S. Lin and D. J. Costello, *Error control coding: Fundamentals and applications*, Prentice-Hall, Englewood Cliffs, NJ, 1983.
3. D. G. Sachs, A. Raghavan, and K. Ramchandran, "Wireless image transmission using multiple-description based concatenated codes," presented at the *Data Compression Conference*, 2000.
4. T. S. Rappaport, *Wireless communications principles and practice*, second edition, Printice Hall, Upper Saddle River, NJ, 2002.
5. K. L. Du and M. N. S. Swamy, *Wireless communication systems: From RF subsystems to 4G enabling technologies*, Cambridge University Press, New York, 2010.
6. M. K. Simon and M. S. Alouini, *Digital communications over fading channles*, second edition, John Wiley & Sons, New York, 2005.
7. E. Biglieri, *Coding for wireless channels*, Springer international edition, New York, 2005.
8. R. C. Gonzalez, *Digital image processing*, second edition, Printice Hall, Upper Saddle River, NJ, 2010.
9. J. Craig and V. Patterson, "Introduction to the practice of telemedicine," *Journal of Telemedicine Telecare*, 2005, 11, pp. 3–9.
10. S. Katzenbeisser and F. A. P. Petitcolas, *Information hiding techniques for steganography and digital watermarking*, Artech House, Inc., Norwood, MA, 2000.

11. H. Abdel-Nabi and A. Al-Haj, "Efficient joint encryption and data hiding algorithm for medical images security," in *Proceedings of 8th International Conference on Information and Communication Systems (ICICS)*, April 2017, pp. 147–152.
12. E. T. Lin and E. J. Delp, "A review of data hiding in digital images," in *Proceedings of the Image Processing, Image Quality, Image Capture Systems Conference (PICS'99)*, June 1999, pp. 274–278.
13. A. Shehab, et al., "Secure and robust fragile watermarking scheme for medical images", *IEEE Access*, 2018, 6, pp. 10269–10278.
14. E. E. Abdallah, *Robust digital watermarking techniques for multimedia protection*, Ph.D thesis, Concordia University, Montreal, QC, March 2009.
15. A. Shaik and V. Thanikaiselvan, "Comparative analysis of integer wavelet transforms in reversible data hiding using threshold based histogram modification," *Journal of King Saud University - Computer and Information Sciences*, 2018.
16. E. Reiter, "Wavelet compression of medical imagery," *Telemedicine Journal*, August 1996, 2(2), pp. 131–137.
17. I. J. Cox, J. Kilian, F. T. Leighton, and T. Shamoon, "Secure spread spectrum watermarking for multimedia," *IEEE Transactions on Image Processing*, December 1997, 6(12), pp. 1673–1687.
18. C. Y. Liu and S. Lin, "Turbo encoding and decoding of Reed-Solomon codes through binary decomposition and self-concatenation," *IEEE Transactions on Communications*, September 2004, 52(9), pp. 1484–1493.
19. C. Berrou and A. Glavieux, "Near optimum error correcting coding and decoding: Turbo codes," *IEEE Transactions on Communications*, October 1996, 44(10), pp. 1261–1271.
20. G. Sherwood and K. Zeger, "Error protection for progressive image transmission over memoryless and fading channels," *IEEE Transactions on Communications*, December 1998, 46(12), pp. 1555–1559.
21. R. Gupta and S. Kumar, "Performance comparison of different forward error correction coding techniques for wireless communication systems," *International Journal of Computer Science and Technology*, September 2011, 2(3), pp. 553–557.
22. G. Mitchell, "Investigation of Hamming, Reed-Solomon and Turbo forward error correcting codes," *ARL-TR-4901*, July 2009, pp. 24.
23. J. Nayak, P. S. Bhat, M. S. Kumar, and R. Acharya, "Reliable and robust transmission and storage of medical images with patient information," in *International Conference on Signal Processing and Communications (SPCOM)*, December 2004, pp. 91–95.
24. P. K. Korrai, M. N. S. Swamy, and K. D. Rao, "Robust transmission of watermarked medical image over wireless channels," in *Proceedings of the IEEE GHTC*, Seattle, WA, Octobet 2012.
25. S. F. Mare, M. Vladutiu, and L. Prodan, "Secret data communication system using steganography, AES and RSA", in *Proceedings of IEEE 17th International Symposium Design and Technology in Electronic Packaging (SIITME)*, October 2011, pp. 339–344.
26. M. S. Sreekutty and P. S. Baiju, "Security enhancement in image steganography for medical integrity verification system," in *Proceedings of International Conference on Circuit, Power and Computing Technologies (ICCPCT)*, April 2017, pp. 1–5.
27. R. Puri and K. Ramchandran, "Multiple description source coding using forward error correcting codes," in *Proceedings of Asilomar Conference on Signals Syststems and Computers* (vol. 1), Pacific Grove, CA, 1999, pp. 342–346.
28. K. Narwal and Y. Sharma, "Performance comparison of Turbo codes with other forward error correcting codes," *International Journal of Electronics and Computer Science Engineering*, 2012, 1(2), pp. 411–415, [Online] www.ijecse.org.

29. B. M. Irany, X. C. Guo, and D. Hatzinakos, "A high capacity reversible multiple watermarking scheme for medical image," in *Proceedings of the IEEE International Conference on DSP*, Corfu, Greece, July 2011, pp. 1–6.

30. Z. Chang and J. Xu, "Reversible run length data embedding for medical Images," in *Proceedings of the IEEE 3rd International Conference on Communication Software and Networks (ICCSN)*, Xi'an, China, May 2011, pp. 260–263.

31. D. Mistry, "Comparison of digital watermarking methods," *International Jouranal Computer Sceince and Engineering*, December 2010, 2(9), pp. 2905–2909.

32. G. Coatrieux, H. Maitre, B. Sankur, B. Rolland, and R. Collorec, "Relevance of watermarking in medical imaging," in *Proceedings of 3rd Conference Information Technology Application in Biomedicine (ITAB)*, Airlington, TX, November 2000, pp. 250–255.

33. E. T. Lin and E. J. Delp, "A review of fragile image watermarks," in *Proceedings of the Multimedia and Security Workshop on Multimedia Contents*, Orlando, FL, October 1999, pp. 25–29.

34. J. Fridrich, "A hybrid watermark for tamper detection in digital images," in *Proceedings of the Fifth International Symposium on Signal Processing and Its Applications*, August 1999, 1, pp.301–304.

35. P. K. Korrai, M. N. S. Swamy, and K. D. Rao, "Performance analysis of a MIMO scheme for watermarked medical images transmission over Rayleigh fading channels," in *Proceedings of the IEEE EMBS Conference*, Langkawi, Malaysia, December 2012.

36. D. Samanta, A. Basu, T. S. Das, V. H. Mankar, A. Ghosh, M. Das, and S. K Sarkar, "SET based logic realization of a robust spatial domain image watermarking," in *Proceedings of 5th International Conference on Electrical and Computer Engineering (ICECE)*, Dhaka, Bangladesh, IEEE, 2008, pp. 986–993.

37. S. P. Mohanty, *Watermarking of digital images*, M.S. thesis, Indian Institute of Science, Bangalore, 1999.

38. N. Memon and P. W. Wong, "Protecting digital media content," *Communications of the ACM*, July 1998, 41(7), pp. 34–43.

39. R. Raturi and A.Kumar, "An analytical approach for health data analysis and finding the correlations of attributes using decision tree and W-logistic modal process," *IJIRCCE*, 2019, 7(6), ISSN (Online): 2320-9801, ISSN (Print): 23209798.

40. M. Jain, R. C. Choudhary, and A. Kumar, "Secure medical image steganography with RSA cryptography using decision tree," in *Proceedings of 2nd International Conference on Contemporary Computer Information (IC3I)*, December 2016, pp. 291–295.

41. J. Kivijarvi, T. Ojala, T. Kaukoranta, A. Kuba, L. Nyul, and O. Nevalainen, "A comparison of lossless compression methods for medical images," *Computerized Medical Imaging and Graphics*, July 1998, 22(4), pp. 323–339.

42. L. Yehia, A. Khedr, and A. Darwish, "Hybrid security techniques for Internet of things healthcare applications," *Advances in Internet of Things*, July 2015, 5, pp. 21–25.

43. M. Elhoseny, G. Ramírez-González, O. M. Abu-Elnasr, S. A. Shawkat, N. Arunkumar, and A. Farouk, "Secure medical data transmission model for IoT-based healthcare systems," *IEEE Access*, 2018, 6, pp. 20596–20608.

44. U. R. Acharya, D. Anand, P. S. Bhat, and U. C. Niranjan, "Compact storage of medical images with patient information," *IEEE Transactions on Information Technology in Biomedicine*, December 2001, 5(4), pp. 320–323.

45. S. P. Mohanty, N. Ranganathan, and R. K. Namballa, "VLSI implementation of invisible digital watermarking algorithms towards the development of a secure JPEG encoder," in *Proceedings of the IEEE Workshop on Signal Processing Systems*, 2003, pp. 183–188.

46. A. Basu, T. S. Das, S. Maiti, N. Islam, and S. K. Sarkar, "FPGA based implementation of robust spatial domain image watermarking algorithm," in *Proceedings of International Conference on Computers and Devices for Communication*, 2009.
47. S. P. Mohanty, K. R. Ramakrishnan, and M. S. Kankanhalli, "A dual watermarking technique for images," in *Proceedings of the 7th ACM International Multimedia Conference* (vol. 2), 1999, pp. 49–51.
48. S. P. Mohanty, N. Ranganathan, and R. K. Namballa, "VLSI implementation of invisible digital watermarking algorithms towards the development of a secure JPEG encoder," in *Proceedings of the IEEE Workshop on Signal Processing Systems*, 2003, pp. 183–188.

12 HCI and Technology Adoption in Healthcare

Neha Mehta and Archana Chaudhary

CONTENTS

12.1 INTRODUCTION TO HCI

The term human–computer interaction (HCI) covers a multidimensional stream of various domains which are emerging from the current designing practices, especially in the domains of health, technology and the industry sector. On the way, the new technologies are providing advancement by incorporating HCI for more and more of their implementation, in order to understand and get exhaustive knowledge about how to adopt HCI and prove it as a boon [1].

The extensive work on HCI was reported in the early 1980s [2], but its roots are found to be established in various disciplines many years earlier. It is a multi-speciality domain for many disciplines but its core is computer and system design. HCI may be classed as an umbrella term that includes various domains of CSCW, i.e. computer-supported collaborative working, CSCR, i.e computer-supported collaborative research, and CSCL, i.e. computer-supported collaborative learning, where each domain is a unchanging subset of the previous one. Historically, HCI has evolved from multiple points resulting in a set of methods towards the set of facts, several methods, theories and certain general abstractions. According to the researchers [3],

> The human–computer interaction is more predominantly defined as a discipline which is concerned with the non-overlapping design, its implementation and evaluation for interactive computing system with human use and also along with the study of various procedures that surrounds them,

HCI seems to be the bridging form of engineering (informatics/computer science) with natural sciences (psychology) and, similarly, usability engineering [4]

DOI: 10.1201/9781003132110-12

is anchored in software technology that supports its implementation. It not only includes an understanding of theories of education, but also incorporates psychology, ergonomics, speech recognition, interfacing, etc. HCI is a difficult endeavour as it needs to be easy, effective and efficient to use, so that interaction in the physical world and virtual world may be embedded in an efficient manner.

The objective of the chapter is to provide a broad view of human–computer interfaces, understanding the nature of human–computer interactions, mechanics, computer systems and interface architecture, along with the evaluation of user interfaces.

12.2 NATURE OF HUMAN–COMPUTER INTERACTIONS

Is it just like the patient in the healthcare waiting room having a thought about how the organisation could be more efficient? Or the patient himself thinking about how to reduce the amount of time spent waiting for the treatment? Or how to work in a healthcare organisation? And how to improve the organisation? The tremendous implications of HCI have paved a way for it. It is about understanding these kinds of situations and using methods and techniques that help in avoiding such problems. It requires a clear technology of how humans interact with machines for providing a solution for the problems. The human brain and machines work in almost similar ways. Human brains have sets of neurons which transmit information through a set of commands and machines utilise AI and ANN (artificial intelligence and artificial neural networks) with fuzzy logic to set commands and transmit through various signals [5].

An organised way towards human recital had begun in earnest at the beginning of the last century with a more targeted emphasis on human manual tasks, and later, impetus was provided to study the interaction between humans and machines by considering a bottom-up approach and top-down approach. These seem to be interchangeable between humans and computers, as in computer machines, the top-down approach is followed from large to small size till the nano level; however, in humans, it has been explored to follow the bottom-up approach by studying unicellular organisms to multicellular organisms in a complex manner and unfolding concepts of signal transmissions. Human interaction happens with the information that is being received and sent through the interacting input device and the interacting output device. When the user interacts with a computer, it gains information in the form of output through the computer machine, and this machine responds by sending the input signal again to the computer machine; then the user's output becomes the machine's input and vice versa (Figure 12.1).

As computers gain popularity and recognition of the interaction between the system and the user grows, concerns about the psychological, theoretical and physical aspects have started becoming widespread. Another domain of research which has a profound effect on human–computer interaction is information science and technology along with the domain of cognitive science and sensors, controlling intelligence and the environment. This system undoubtedly utilises an interdisciplinary and multidisciplinary approach by incorporating inputs from all disciplines. It is in alignment with the human body, towards acquiring a deep

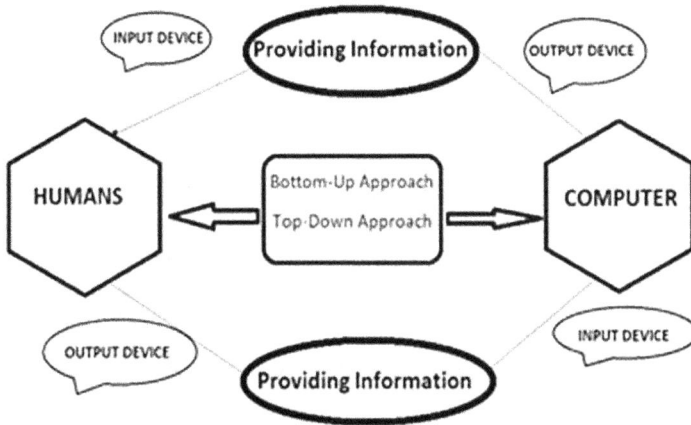

FIGURE 12.1   Input becoming output in HCI utilising both bottom-up and top-down approaches.

knowledge of the body in order to understand its functioning in response to stimulus (external or internal) by getting expertise in understanding the metabolism. However, the physiology behind this is again a complex web of events going on in the human body. In computers, there is also a need for a stream for getting the users' cognitive, perceptual and problem-solving skills towards users' physical capabilities and their abilities for understanding the wider context of interaction. To make human–computer interaction effective, inputs are required from all the dimensions in order to make it more accessible, useable and applicable for the entire population.

The human brain acts as an information processor, which receives inputs from the outside world, stores that information, manipulates it and thus uses this information along with reacting towards the information that has been received. However, machines have their input and output devices (such as keyboards, touch boards, speech inputs, LCD screens, head-mounted displays) from where information is processed in the processing unit. The information is received through the different senses, like sight, hearing capabilities and touching. These are stored in the desired system memory, as random access memory (RAM), or permanently in long-term memory as magnetic and optical disks in machines. It can then be used in problem-solving. The recurrent familiar situations promote people to access and apply their basic developmental skills in that domain, as their information structures become more accurate. The interface designer in HCI should remain conscious of the properties of the devices within the assembled system [6, 7]. This includes not only input/output devices, but each and every aspect that has an influence on the behaviour of the interface since all of this affects the basic style of the interaction in progress. Human perception and cognition are generally found to be complex and sophisticated , though they are never without limitations, so computers and HCI need to be explored more to understand the interaction more efficiently.

12.3 ARCHITECTURE OF HCI

The HCI incorporate various tools and insights from many fields, including robotics, control systems, data mining, speech and face recognition, probability, operation research, cognitive science and neuroscience, and computer science in the core. HCI is not merely about the designing of software or creating devices but it is an interaction through a proper framework, focusing on understanding the situation, changes and environment and how the user deals with them as every individual is different in its own way. The architecture of HCI should be such that it helps in developing interventions in all the varying situations by using different techniques including software, the web and various physical devices. Currently, we are simulating human intelligence through which the interpretation can be simulated, replaced, extended, or expanded in intelligence through HCI. However, researchers have reported the need for focussing on new extreme heights through the development of cutting-edge technologies such as a brain–computer interface which is going to be the future of HCI [8]. The architecture of HCI focuses on the range of activities that involves the machine with the user and is implemented in three domains, notably physical, cognitive and affective.

The physical technologies are designed on relative human senses: including audible, visible and touch. The vision-based devices are either switch-based or may be the pointing devices for input and visual or printing for the output. However, the devices for audition need to be more advanced and require sophisticated speech recognition in order to facilitate the interaction between humans and computers. They include speech signals and/or messages which are produced as output by machines in the form of output signals. Examples include the beeps or navigation commands of a GPS device. The haptic devices [9], which are responsible for interfacing to generate sensations in the skin and muscles, are reported as complicated and comparatively costlier. They are generally made for virtual reality or disability assistive applications. Recently, advanced technologies [10] along with former methods, have used networking and animation to design wearable or wireless devices or virtual devices. Examples of such devices are GPS navigating systems, military devices (e.g. thermal vision, tracking movements using GPS and/or environmental scanning), radio frequency identification (RFID) products, personal digital assistants and virtual tours for real estate business, etc.

For attaining good architecture, the cognitive aspect forms a main perspective on users about who they are, whether it remembers that they are different or not and trying to imagine their likes and dislikes. The universal structure of the application is also important to understand these materials. In the case of interaction design, these materials include not only the technical devices (input and output devices), but also humans. If human treatment is required in design with minimal care as physical objects, then it is clear that after accidents "human errors" would be "design error". The design is always developed by understanding the interaction deeply between humans and computers and also considering their limitations, as we have to make a room for those errors. The human factors in the adoption and implementation of innovation play an important role in the architectural design of a machine. An adoption-based focus in the initial phases and ultimately in implementation, according to these authors [10], may help in preventing the various forms of resistance and thus reducing the levels of criticism and frustration while designing.

The architecture for HCI is iterative and never complete as it explores the breadth of technology application, current and emerging trends and has more advanced control paradigms. HCI utilises design thinking to handle understanding design, prototyping, and evaluation as well as specific topic areas within human–computer interaction including ubiquitous and social computing.

12.3.1 System Architecture

The configuration of its design plays a crucial role in the system architecture. The system architecture of HCI incorporates the number of interfaces, which are made to accomplish the entire task through the diversity of both of its inputs and outputs. When any one modality is used in the system, then it is called a uni-modal system. That may be further divided into the following categories:

1. Visual dependent
2. Audio dependent
3. Sensor dependent

The uni-modal HCI system on the basis of its modality has got its application in the various categories of visual HCI, like the tracking of different body parts, recognition of the body gesture, tracking of the eye movement, analysis of facial expressions and many more. The modalities serve for the direct interaction between the human and the computer. In the category of audio HCI, the interaction is done through the audio signals. In contrast to the minute variation in the visual signals, the audio signals are referred to as the most trustable and unique information providers. The different categories of application in audio HCI are in recognition of speaker voices, speech voices, analysis of auditory emotional voice, laugh-cry sound detection, etc. More research in this field [11, 12] is helpful in identifying typical speech pitch and auditory signs. However, the sensor-based modality is the combination of different physical sensors to be used between the machine and the user. Such a kind of HCI is sophisticated to be used. The examples in this modality include mouse-based interaction, keyboard-based interaction, usage of haptic on pressure sensors, joysticks, etc. Another is a multimodal-based HCI system; in this system, the multiple modalities are combined. There is a creation of a multimodal interface, which is the combination of two or more modes and goes beyond the mouse and the keyboard. It may be the combination of different speech signals, body gestures, facial expressions, etc. Due to its versatility in usage and the combination of more than the conventional type of modalities, the multimodel system has got its application in the domains that are listed as follows:

- Towards the creation of intelligent homes and offices
- Towards the creation of intelligent games

- Towards disabled society
- Towards e-commerce
- Towards video conferencing, and many more

12.4   INTERACTION MECHANICS WITH ACTIVITIES INVOLVED

The HCI involves interaction mechanics along with the activities to increase usability and make them more effective and efficient along with user satisfaction. The user does not see themselves as devices in a machine but interestingly wants to use it for a better work environment and wants to enjoy what they are doing. HCI focus on ergonomics, aesthetics, economics, legality and safety in the context of the physical environment. Interactivity is the core of all upcoming modern interfaces and plays a never-ending role. After looking at an interface, it is presumed that along with a focus on the visually different parts (like menus, text, options, formatting, more choices), the dynamics, the way they react towards a user's actions, should also be considered, obviously in a low manner. In earlier HCI systems [13], the order of interaction was usually evaluated by the machine but now a focus is also there on the users' understanding and knowledge. The interaction between humans and machines doesn't happen in isolation but is also affected by various social, organisational and environmental factors. These factors can influence the effectiveness of the interaction as they are somehow beyond the designers' control. However, they may be limited by providing awareness to the designers in advance.

The effective strategies for designing HCI helps in building interactive systems which provide different paradigms for the designing and application of usable interactive systems. The input of creative designing can never be replaced but may be exploited, but it always poses a benefit by repeating its paybacks in one way or the other in multiple different designs. The repeated use may sometimes not provide authenticity but provides a complementary approach, which strengthens the development of a theory to support the paradigm for its application being repeated.

12.5   HCI AS STATE OF THE ART

HCI has got its present form by adopting various advancements and techniques happening parallel in many scientific areas, intercepting each other, which include artificial intelligence, data science, fuzzy logic, artificial neural networks, speech recognition, etc. To get a major breakthrough in HCI all aspects of interactions have been explored and utilised as per timely specifications. As in humans, the sensory system plays a significant role in interacting with nature; similarly, in human–computer interaction, the sensory devices have brought revolutionary changes making HCI more efficient and productive. As a consequence, HCI is increasingly driving towards adopting those frameworks which have a multimodal approach and uses information exchanges via natural sensory modes which utilise one simultaneously or in combination for sight, or building information modelling (BIM) and touch senses. Humans being employed as the central burden for the interaction needs to be explored more by considering other attributes such as attitude, perception, mood and emotion. So, the role of multimodal modalities needs to be explored in depth for establishing a framework which enhances the application of HCI in today's scenario.

Machine learning plays a pervasive role in human life; with the advent of information systems, humans started interacting for enhancing scientific research, advancement, technology and knowledge. The human–machine interaction provides a major breakthrough when it enters the health and military sectors searching for information, research and advancement. Now after involving other elements from diverse fields of science and humanity the interaction between humans and machines gains new heights. The diverse fields utilise not only subfields of computer science and engineering but are also focussed on psychology, ergonomics, cognitive science, etc. This new paradigm shift has brought a revolutionary change in society. This was due to understanding human nature in all aspects including emotions and perception along with a better understanding of interactions between humans, computers and the environment.

HCI utilises interface through modern sensory inputs and output devices ranging from pointers to face recognition. As interface plays a significant role, all success depends on how you provide input or receive output through a machine, for example, in the case of utilising robots in operation theatres. HCI has a dependency on interface design for efficient processing, and humans being the main element plays a crucial role in it. So, interfacing devices should be user-friendly, easily accessible and flexible as per the environment and may be customised as per the requirement. The major constraint in this is to provide awareness and popularity so that it may gain popularity making ease for those using it.

The human–computer interaction (HCI) field has lots of growth and development in different lines to be more economically and technologically crucial and popular. It utilises various architects for interface designing, multimodal processing, intelligent and smart input and output sensory devices. The design should be considered intelligently and smartly in order to make it more active rather than passive.

12.6 FACTORS INVOLVED IN THE ADOPTION OF TECHNICAL INNOVATION

The HCI utilises technologies that are based on safety-specific software applications, building information modelling, ICT modelling, and many more. However, wearable technologies are still not adapted fully and are in their initial stages in terms of technology advancement. The currently lacking synchronised, efficient and integrated systems [14] are some of the drivers which need to be focused on for HCI utilisation.

There are several different routes for supporting the technology adoption in this domain on the basis of factors that are responsible for adopting technical innovation including the reluctance to be changed by the stakeholders. Due to the cutting-edge technologies, the common resistance that is faced towards construction and uncertainty about practical benefits of new technologies are turned out as a challenge that impedes the development and implementation of the innovative technologies. Understanding the psychological factors that drive technology adoption in the public interest is a part of success for the influence of factors psychologically. They may be overcome by motivating the utilisation of new technologies and justifying the cost–time benefits and low energy consumptions which play a significant role in the successful completion of design projects. Another consideration is the adoption of technology by users; their consent is expected for the benefits to be obtained. Accepting new tools results in unplanned changes in the manner of how these tasks are performed, which impacts the users, so individual factors also play a significant role which is referred to as individuals' cognitive interpretations of innovation and themselves. Social factors also play an important role in the adoption of HCI; however, the support system plays a major role in overcoming it. Although, the technical respect of this application of the technology may be challenging for some users, which may be overcome by addressing the technical knowledge in training sessions for its successful implementation. There is always an enormous amount of potential for the emerging research and its impact of social influence for the adoption of technology, in every context, where usage is a relatively new behaviour of adoption.

HCI may be utilised to its fullest by having a more practically oriented approach by integrating new technologies and proper support systems to identify and understand the problem and developing it as per the user's perspective.

REFERENCES

1. Karat, J., & Karat, C.-M. (2003). The evolution of user-centered focus in the human-computer interaction field. *IBM Systems Journal*, *42*(4), 532–541.
2. Gould, J. D., & Lewis, C. (1985). Designing for usability: Key principles and what designers think. *Communications of the ACM*, *28*, 300–311.
3. Dominic, P. D. D., Jati, H., Sellappan, P., & Nee, G. K. (2011). A comparison of Asian e-government websites quality: Using a non-parametric test. *International Journal of Business Information Systems*, *7*(2), 220–246.
4. Kuniavsky, M. (2010). *Smart things: Ubiquitous computing user experience design*. Burlington, MA: Morgan Kaufmann.
5. Hancock, P. A., Pepe, A. A., & Murphy, L. L. (2005). Hedonomics: The power of positive and pleasurable ergonomics. *Ergonomics Design*, *13*(1), 8–14.
6. Chung, W., & Fortier, S. (2013). Context as a system, product as a component, and the relationship as experience. In A. Marcus (Ed.), *Design, user experience, and usability: Design philosophy, methods, and tools* (Vol. 8012, pp. 29–37). Las Vegas, NV: Springer.
7. Fitts, P. M. (1954). The information capacity of the human motor system in controlling the amplitude of movement. *Journal of Experimental Psychology*, *47*(6), 381.
8. Dalgleish, T., & Power, M. J. (2000). *Handbook of cognition and emotion*. London, UK: John Wiley & Sons Ltd.
9. Kemeny, M. E., & Shestyuk, A. (2010). Emotions, the neuroendocrine and immune systems and health. In M. Lewis, J. M. Haviland-Jones, & L. F. Barrett (Eds.), *Handbook of emotions* (3rd ed, pp. 661–665). New York: The Guilford Press.
10. Hussain, A., Abdullah,A., Husni, H., & Mkpojiogu, E. O. C. (2016). Interaction design principles for edutainment systems: Enhancing the communication skills of children with autism spectrum disorders. *Revista Tecnica de la Facultad de Ingenieria Universidad del Zulia*, *39*(8), 45–50.
11. Hussain, A., Mkpojiogu, E. O. C., Musa, J., Mortada, S., & Yue, W. S. (2018). Mobile experience evaluation of an e-Reader app. *Journal of Telecommunication, Electronic & Computer Engineering (JTEC)*, *10*(1–10), 11–15.

12. Jokela, T., Laine, J., & Nieminen, M. (2013). Usability in RFP's: The current practice and outline for the future human-computer interaction. In M. Kurosu (Ed.), *Applications and services* (pp. 101–106). Springer.
13. Raturi, R., & Kumar, A. (2019). An analytical approach for health data analysis and finding the correlations of attributes using decision tree and W-logistic modal process. *IJIRCCE*, 7(6), ISSN (Online): 2320-9801, ISSN (Print): 23209798.
14. Chandrasekaran, S., & Kumar, A. (2018). Implementing medical data processing with Ann with hybrid approach of implementation. *Journal of Advanced Research in Dynamical and Control Systems – JARDCS, 10*, 45–52.

13 A Comparative and Comprehensive Analysis of Prediction of Parkinson's Disease

N. Prasath, Vigneshwaran Pandi, Sindhuja Manickavasagam, Prabu Ramadoss and S. Subha

CONTENTS

13.1 INTRODUCTION

Parkinson's disease may be a liberal neurodegenerative illness characterised by inactive tremor, akinesia, rigidity, bradykinesia and postural unpredictability, produced by the discerning collapse of dopaminergic nerve cells inside the nucleus niger, leading to lower dopamine levels within the brain. Mutations within the glucocerebrosidase gene constitute the only large risk factor for the event of sporadic paralysis agitans. An environmental factor for Parkinson's includes drinking groundwater and consuming manganese. Another common divisor for Parkinson's is identified as Lewy bodies. Lewy bodies (protein clumps) cover cells in the brain, interfering with their functions. Cramped handwriting, uncontrollable movements while sleeping, limb stiffness, voice changes, rigid countenance or masking and stooped posture are all early signs of Parkinson's disease. Also, disturbance of memory and thinking ability may be a non-motor symptom related to Parkinson's. Many of us with Parkinson's disease feel distracted or disorganised, or have difficulty planning and completing tasks. To begin, based on the assessment of the relationship between GBA mutation status and neuropsychological outcomes, the status of GBA mutation may be an independent risk factor for cognitive impairment in patients with PD, CDR (Clinical Dementia Rating) and clinical diagnoses [1]. Patients of Ashkenazi-Jewish origin with Parkinson's disease were also screened for seven founder GBA mutations,

DOI: 10.1201/9781003132110-13

and the findings revealed that for both moderate and severe heterozygous individuals, the risk and AAO (age at onset) of Parkinson's disease were increased. GBA mutations were differentially affected, which had important implications for guidance [2]. A multitask diffusion adaptation strategy with mixture weights, accompanied by simulation of connectivity in the brain and applying intensities, is used to distinguish between normal and abnormal brain functions. The findings show that multitask learning approaches are often used to improve brain communication patterns [3]. An SVM (support vector machine—to describe the tradeoff between training set error minimisation and margin maximisation) to accurately predict Parkinson's disease, assisted by bacterial foraging optimisation (BFO), was developed. This achieved optimal generalisation ability while preventing overfitting and defined the key parameters for effective prediction [4]. Asynchronous detection supported deep brain stimulation was wont to monitor the patient's hand movements. The results produce a difference between the working of the left and right hemispheres [5]. Additionally, the wearable sensor was wont to record the daily activity and this was mainly utilised in a lifestyle environment. For physical activities, the experiment yields time quantity analyses [6]. A common method of evaluating postural instability in Parkinson's disease patients is the pull test (a tug on the patient's shoulders). It considers ten parameters in order to move the centre of gravity away from the neutral position. The findings were used to build a ROC graph and to categorise patients [7]. To supply patients with effective exercises and to enhance their posture stability SBS rehabilitation of dynamic weight shifting mechanisms was used. It detects the postures and tent of patients during their course and provides feedback to enhance the steadiness [8].

13.2 RELATED WORKS

A. H. Hadjahmadi et al. [9] proposed a classification-based emotionally supportive network for the determination of Parkinson's disease. In Parkinson's disease, the problem conjointly ordinarily causes a speed or freeze of development. Regression, support vector machines (SVM), classification and regression trees (CART), Bayesian network, and artificial neural networks were all used in the proposed framework (ANN). Ali Saad et al. [10] proposed a Bayesian belief network for detecting infected patients and customs a motion dataset obtained from real Parkinson's disease patients who were walking at the time and had real change times. Each document was created using a framework that included estimating facts from the three sensors in order to determine whether or not climate freezing of gait (FoG) occurred. S. Amit et al. [11] investigated a system for grouping and sorting Parkinson's patients based on their postural response using an L2 standard measurement linked to support vector machines and 24 patients were examined. Every patient languished following investigation convention of the assessment of their property stability: beginning, eyes open on force stage and second, eyes open on foam put on force stage (FO). Aprajita Sharma et al. [12] proposed fake neural organisation, design acknowledgement and a backing vector machine. It is acclimated provision the specialists inside the assignment of Parkinson's disease. Arvind Kumar Tiwari [13] proposed the premier significant component among every one of the highlights to foresee Parkinson's disease.

The changed AI-based techniques like sacking, boosting, arbitrary backwoods, revolution woods, irregular subspace, SVM, multilayer perceptron and decision tree–based strategies are wont to anticipate the loss of motion agitans. Athanasios Tsanas et al. [14] proposed how precisely the new algorithms are used to favour PD subjects from healthy controls. From continued vowels, there are a total of 132 dysphonia steps. Four feature selection algorithms are used to pick and two statistical classifiers, random forests and support vector machines are used to map a binary classification answer. This method makes use of an existing database that includes 263 samples from 43 subjects. The new dysphonia measurements with ten dysphonia features performed well and achieved an accuracy of 99% in classification.

Chen et al. [15] developed two methodologies, the nested-RF and nested-SVM classifiers, that can search for the model's ideal boundaries naturally. Five datasets of malignant growth (brain cancer, carcinoma, DLBCL, leukaemia and prostate cancer) and one of the proposed classifiers' output were evaluated using a dataset of illnesses. In loss of motion agitans characterisation, the nested-SVM classifier showed better execution with exactness up to 93 out of 200, an incredible outcome from three elective classifiers. The forecast model tree-based characterisation was proposed by Azad et al. [16]. The classical decision tree, ID3 and choice stumps, a term suggested, are used for preparing and determining the feasibility of different symptoms that contribute to Parkinson's disease, such as tremors in the legs, arms and hands, disabled discourse clarity and developmental problems. Bouchikhi et al. [17] suggested artificial neural networks (ANN), neural data mining, regression and decision trees for a powerful dataset to distinguish healthy people from those with Parkinson's disease. For successfully finding datasets to isolate healthy individuals and lack of motion agitans, artificial neural networks (ANN), neural knowledge handling, regression and decision trees were used. A. Chen et al. [18] proposed the nested–random forest (nested-RF) and nested–support vector machine (nested-SVM) classifiers for the prediction of five malignancy datasets (cerebrum disease, carcinoma, DLBCL, leukaemia, prostate malignant growth) and one illness dataset (Parkinson's). A. H. Chen et al. [19] introduced two methodologies, the nested-RF classifier and the nested-SVM classifier, that can search for the model's ideal boundaries naturally. We apply these classifiers to five malignant growths (mind malignant growth, DLBCL, prostate malignant growth, colon malignant growth and leukaemia) as well as Parkinson's disease to see how successful they are. Using the ANOVA consistency determination technique, the major qualities were selected from those with a P value of less than 0.05. After analysing the characterisation results obtained from four different classifiers, the proposed nested-SVM classifier is shown to be the best one. The nested-SVM classifier outperforms the other three classifiers by around 2–5% in terms of grouping execution (exactness, affectability and explicitness) when applied to five malignancy datasets. H. Chen et al. [20] suggested an FKNN-based system in relation to support vector machines (SVM)-based methodologies for a dataset containing 31 biomedical voice estimations from 23 Parkinson's disease patients. The FKNN-based framework's highest order precision (96.07%), obtained using a ten-crease cross approval strategy, will ensure a solid analytic model for Parkinson infection position. The proposed structure by C. Cho et al. [21] combines a calculation joining principal component analysis (PCA) with linear discriminant analysis (LDA). It suggested a step-by-step examination framework for locating a walking example of Parkinson's disease misuse of computer vision. S. G. Farhad et al. [22] introduced an MLP, RBF and ANN-based method to distinguish between clinical factors of tests (N = 195). MLP and RBF characterisation exactness for the knowledge set was 93.22% and 86.44%, respectively. To predict behaviour related to quake starting, D. Wu et al. [23] proposed a radial basis function neural network (RBFNN) assisted particle swarm optimisation (PSO) and principal component analysis (PCA) with local field potential (LFP) information reported by means of the incitement anodes. To distinguish healthy individuals from those with Parkinson's disease, H. Hazan et al. [24] proposed the subtractive clustering features in a kernel-based extreme learning machine weighting methodology (CFW-KELM).

Hung Nguyen et al. [6] proposed a calculation to handle the information from the inertial estimation unit in order to identify and fragment unstructured ADL in people with Parkinson's disease (PD) in a free-living setting. The proposed methodology allowed for the precise location of 1,610 ADL events conducted by nine local-area-abiding older adults with PD in a recreated free-living environment with 90% precision (affectability = 90.8%, explicitness = 97.8%), thus portioning these exercises within 350 milliseconds of the "best quality standard" manual division. These findings demonstrated the potential for the proposed technique to be used to spontaneously discern and segment ADL in people with Parkinson's disease in a free-living environment in the long run. Indira et al. [25] suggested a natural AI approach and established the Parkinson's disease for the benefit of the individual's discourse/voice. The developer used a fluffy C-implied bunch and example recognition-based approach to distinguish between sound and Parkinson's disease–affected people. To distinguish loss of motion agitans from sound topics, J. Rusz et al. [26] propose to find the simplest blend of estimations, and an implemented support vector machine was suggested. This system prompts an 85% general grouping execution. In fact, we've discovered ties between correspondence and explanation proportions and bradykinesia and unbending nature in Parkinson's disease. T. Kapoor et al. [27] suggested that MFCC and VQ acknowledge debate. The MFCC employs discourse examination outlines in relation to the recurrence space, and the vector division was chosen as the codebook with the least twisting. The 20 phonations are used in daily conversation and in patients with Parkinson's disease. In the 90th and 95th classifiers, respectively, in the customary voice and voice of Parkinson's disorder rate, vector division results with a codebook. The discretisation strategy, help vector machines, C4.5, the k-closest neighbours technique, and naive Bayes are more tasteful techniques that are wont to group the dataset, suggested by E. Kaya et al. [28]. The dataset was organised using discretised and non-discretised judgements, implying that discretisation can be used to attribute a loss of motion agitans.

Using each of the 22 highlights and a parallel choice class ("0" is solid and "1" is IPD choice class), Kenneth Revett et al. [29] proposed jitter, sparkle, important, music/commotion proportions, enlightening measurements and correlational elements (non-straight powerful examination). A legendary animal and disarray structure were created to appear at the precision of the grouping technique, and the research partners' degreed instructing attempt was characterised. The probability of exactness is 100%. Khemphila et al. [30] suggested a multi-layer perceptron (MLP) with a backpropagation learning calculation that could be used to evaluate Parkinson's disease effectively (PD). The specialist's knowledge and expertise completed the discovery. However, there have been cases of incorrect assignment and treatment reported by territory units. The patients' area has demanded that a range of tests be needed for assignment. In certain cases, not all of the tests are helpful in determining the cause of an illness. The patients' assignments were acclimated by the engineered neural organisation zone. B. K. Kihel et al. [31] suggested CLONCLAS and probabilistic neural network (PNN) as tools for distinguishing between healthy and Parkinson's-affected patients (PAP). We strive to steal accommodating properties like programmed acknowledgement, memorisation and transformation by taking inspiration from the usual invulnerable frameworks. CLONCLAS was fascinated by the algorithmic standards that were developed based on the measurement of training medication.

Korosh Rouhollahi et al. [32] proposed a closed-loop control framework to invigorate two zones of BG all the while. The oddity of the proposed regulator structure is twofold: an initial AFEL/PSF regulator and a second concurrent incitement of GPi and STN. To convey reasonable stimulatory control signs to the cerebrum, a closed-loop control framework with criticism is utilised from a hand quake. Thus, the quake has a direct connection to stimulatory energy force. As a result, the stimulatory energy capacity is drastically decreased. We were able to reduce the computational time and increase the information set by combining fluffy entropy-based component choice with a closeness classifier, as proposed by P. Luukka et al. [33]. To gather data, a variety of drug voice estimates from healthy people and people with Parkinson's disease were used (PD). For the Parkinson infection dataset, C. Ma et al. [34] suggested a completely new crossover technique called kernel-based extreme learning machine with subtractive clustering features weighting (SCFWKELM), which basically beats SVM, KNN and extreme learning machine (ELM) approaches. Mehmet Can et al. [35] suggested an equal distributed neural organisation of a couple of hidden layers, to identify people with traditional vocal signs and Parkinson's disease symptoms. Caglar et al. [36] proposed using ANNs, multilayer perceptron (MLP) and radial basis function (RBF) networks, as well as an adaptive neuro-fuzzy classifier (ANFC) with phonetic fences to distinguish healthy people with individual palladium. The least challenging acknowledgement findings came from a versatile neuro-fuzzy classifier with etymological help. For grouping healthy and Parkinson's patients, Shahbakhi et al. [37] used a genetic algorithm (GA) and a support vector machine (SVM). F0 (major recurrence or pitch), jitter, gleam and commotion-to-sound proportion, which are all essential factors for voice signal, were all upheld by voice flags. Chen et al. [15] developed dual methodologies, nested-RF and nested-SVM classifiers, that can look for the model's ideal boundaries in a natural way. To evaluate the presentation of the proposed classifiers, five datasets of malignancy (mind disorder, colon malignancy, DLBCL, leukaemia and prostate disease) and one dataset of illness (Parkinson's) were used. In the grouping of Parkinson's disease, the nested-SVM classifier had a stronger presentation with a precision of more than 93, which was 200th, an incredible result from the elective three classifiers.

Naive Bayes, feature selection naive Bayes (FSNB), correlation-based feature selection naive Bayes (CFS-NB) and support vector machines (SVM) were proposed by D. A. Morales et al. [38]. Geetha Ramani et al. [39] suggested a number of data mining methods, including SVM, KNN, random tree, partial least square regression (PLS) and so on to predict dataset medication voice estimations from 31 individuals, 23 of whom had Parkinson's disease (PD). The calculations for higher characterisation of purpose were added to the sifting, with the most modest number of characteristics for which the better order was selected and achieved. C. Nivedita et al. [40] suggested an artificial neural network (ANN) with backpropagation to group neurodegenerative problems with side effects in a consistent manner. There are six distinct types of clinical side effects associated with neurodegenerative diseases. Problems such as memory, communication, personality changes, odd behaviours, lack of willful control and standard medical problems are all common. PC-assisted determination (CADx) systems were introduced by A. Ozcift et al. [41] to increase precision. To polygenic uncertainty, heart, and Parkinson's datasets, random forest (RF) aggregate classifiers of 30 AI algorithmic guidelines were used, including correlation-based feature selection (CFS) calculation and decision tree forecast. Prashanth et al. [42] proposed support vector machine (SVM) and factory loss data from the 40-item University of Pennsylvania Smell Identification Test (UPSIT) and sleep behaviour data from the rapid eye development Rest Behavior Disorder Screening structure (RBDSQ) from the Parkinson's Progression Markers Initiative (PPMI) data collection were used to create decision tree strategies.

Przybyszewski et al. [43] suggested the development lines in the stage space are plotted reflexive saccades estimations. To predict medicine voice estimates from 31 participants, 23 of whom had lost motion agitans, Geetha Ramani et al. [44] proposed a variety of information-mining approaches such as SVM, KNN, random tree, partial least square regression (PLS) and so on. The smallest number of characteristics for which the higher characterisation was selected and achieved was added to the calculations for higher-order purposes. Resul Das et al. [39] suggested neural organisations, knowledge preparation and neural networks. A relative report on the loss of motion agitans informational index was generated using neural investigation, multivariate analysis and decision trees. The procedure was assigned to Parkinson's disease and upheld the SAS code, according to the characterisation. R. N. Alcalay et al. [45] involved CORE-PD participants who were tested for PARKIN, LRRK2 and GBA transformations and were given a neuropsychological battery, while those who were tested for PARKIN, LRRK2 and GBA transformations were given a University of Pennsylvania Smell Identification Test (UPSIT). There were 33 GBA transition transporters and 60 noncarriers with some inherited transformation among the group's members. Essential tests were carried out on 26 GBA heterozygous shift transporters without extra transformations and 39 noncarriers with age and PD terms coordinated. Changed z-scores of individual neuropsychological assessments were used to establish five psychological areas: psychomotor speed, consideration, memory, visuospatial ability and leader work. Clinical analyses (normal, mild cognitive impairment [MCI], dementia) were classified as incognisant in terms of genotypes based on neuropsychological execution and utilitarian hindrance as measured by the

Clinical Dementia Rating (CDR) ranking. GBA transition status was investigated in relation to neuropsychological execution, CDR, and clinical decisions. A. Rubén et al. [1] suggested five different grouping criteria based on a covering highlight option plan that is capable of predicting all of the classification variables with an accuracy range of 72–92%. Furthermore, grouping into the three main seriousness classifications (gentle, moderate and extreme) was incorporated into polarity problems, in which paired classifiers outperform single classifiers and choose different subsets of non-engine manifestations.

The expectation maximisation (EM) calculation was proposed by A. Saad et al. [46], who proposed a method for learning a probabilistic graphical model by itself, the Bayesian belief network (BBN), which is a network of Bayesian beliefs. Voice and penmanship are used to forecast a blended procurement arrangement with electronic pen and discourse signals. Based on the investigation of voice and penmanship, this paper predicts collection. L. Salhi et al. [3] proposed a method for extracting an element vector from discourse tests using wavelet analysis; after that, a multilayer neural network (MNN), a three-layer feed-forward network with sigmoid actuation, and a backpropagation algorithm (BPA) classifier were used. For reverberation images, Salvatore et al. [47] proposed to predict individual differential conclusions of Parkinson's disease; a controlled AI calculation based on principal components analysis as a highlight extraction method and support vector machines were used (PD), as well as a progressive supranuclear palsy (PSP) MRI dataset. The proposed arrangement of obsessive voice from typical voice by V. Sellam et al. [48] uses a support vector machine (SVM) and radial basis function neural network (RBFNN) in the implementation of RBFNN. Adolescent voices, both regular and neurotic, are accustomed to training and researching classifiers. The discourse signal was then dissected to identify acoustic boundaries including signal energy, pitch and formant frequencies. T. Sriram et al. [5] applied random forest, KNN, naive Bayes and support vector machine voice to the dataset for lack of motion against the class segment "status", which was set to zero for happiness and one for metal. Bocklet et al. [49] suggested an SVM- and correlation-based characterisation of Parkinson's disease's impact on an individual's discourse/speech. Parkinson's disease was recognised using verbalisation, voice and prosodic assessments. A. Tsanas et al. [50] suggested a sign approach using a non-linear method with a large dataset (dataset is voice/discourse reported without the need for a doctor in the clinic) distributed over a large area to measure discourse signal. It checked the perceivability of successive, faraway, real, precise UPDRS telemonitoring based on self-managed discourse tests and conducted abuse nonlinear relapse and order recipes.

X. Wan et al. [51] proposed three relative investigations intended to assess the presentation of MegaSNPHunter. The primary research relies on manufactured data obtained from epistasis models. The following one is focused on a genome-wide analysis of Parkinson's disease (information procured by utilising Illumina HumanHap300 SNP chips). The third one selects the rheumatoid joint inflammation concentrate from the Wellcome Trust Case Control Consortium (WTCCC) using the Affymetrix GeneChip 500K Mapping Array Collection. MegaSNPHunter outperforms the competition and announces a slew of planned collaborations for the two genuine tests. D. Wu et al. [52] proposed a radial basis function neural network (RBFNN) in light of particle swarm optimisation (PSO) and principal component analysis with local field potential (LFP) information recorded by means of the incitement anodes to foresee movement identified with quake beginning. LFPs from the subthalamic nucleus (STN) gotten through profound cerebrum cathodes embedded in a Parkinson's patient are utilised to prepare the organisation. Electromyographic (EMG) signals from the patient's lower arm were captured in conjunction with LFPs to control quake events, which are then compared to the organisation's display. It has been discovered that precise position accuracy of up to 89% is possible. Execution correlations between a standard RBFNN and an RBFNN based on PSO have also been performed, showing a slight reduction in execution but a large reduction in computational overhead. Z. Cai et al. [23] suggested that an optimal support vector machine (SVM) be set up in view of bacterial foraging optimisation (BFO) to effectively predict PD. On the basis of a PD informational selection based on vocal estimations, the feasibility of the proposed technique, BFO-SVM, was accepted. The proposed technique and two of the most commonly used boundary advancement techniques were compared to an SVM based on the structure quest strategy and an SVM based on particle swarm optimisation. Furthermore, to increase forecast accuracy, the help highlight determination was used before the BFO-SVM technique, resulting in the RF-BFO-SVM being proposed. The results showed that the system worked extremely well in terms of arrangement execution, with an average order exactness of 97.42%. Ziv Gan-Or et al. [4] dissected 1,000 Ashkenazi-Jewish patients with PD for seven organisers, for GBA transformations and guided a meta-analysis of danger and AAO according to GBA genotype (serious or gentle change). The research included 11,453 patients with Parkinson's disease and 14,565 healthy controls from the general population. The factual investigation was completed with and without progression modification (steady or observational), taking into account inclinations that may have influenced the results.

Zhennao Cai et al. [2] proposed a technique, a transformative-based knowledge method named CBFO-FKNN, which was created by linking the chaotic bacterial foraging optimisation (CBFO) through the Gaussian change method with FKNN. The FKNN's boundary tuning problems were effectively resolved by integrating the CBFO technique. The proposed CBFO-FKNN was thoroughly compared to the PD datasets in terms of order exactness, affectability, particularity and AUC (region under the recipient working trademark bend). The method outperformed five other models based on BFO, particle swarm optimisation, genetic calculations, natural product fly streamlining and firefly calculation, as well as three advanced AI strategies including support vector machine (SVM), SVM with nearby learning-based part option and machine learning, in a tenfold cross-approval. Indrajit Mandal et al. [53] using a robust inference method, suggested an improved diagnosis prediction accuracy for Parkinson's disease (PD) to avoid patient delays and misdiagnosis. The proposed system used metrics for determining prediction accuracy such as specificity, sensitivity, accuracy and other observable parameters. Using linear logistic regression and sparse multinomial logistic regression, this proposed scheme achieved the highest accuracy of 100%, 0.983 in sensitivity and 0.996 in specificity.

The sparse multinomial logistic regression, random forest ensemble with support vector machines and principal components analysis, artificial neural networks and boosting methods are all used in the robust inference system.

Gunjan Pahuja et al. [54] commented that on the benchmark (voice) dataset, they proposed three types of classifiers, namely multilayer perceptron, support vector machine, and K-nearest neighbour, which were discussed to compare and determine which of these classifiers is the most effective and accurate for PD classification. The main challenge of prediction of PD is identifying the most appropriate classification algorithm on a local dataset. D. Ahmadi Rastegar et al. [55] proposed using serum samples from a clinically well-characterised longitudinally followed Michael J. Fox Foundation cohort of PD patients with and without the common leucine-rich repeat kinase 2 (LRRK2) G2019S mutation to suggest a prediction of PD progression. The best prediction models for the motor symptom severity scales, with NRMSE of 0.1123 for the Hoehn and Yahr scale and 0.1193 for the Unified Parkinson's Disease Rating Scale part three (UPDRS III), were found using the normalised root mean square error (NRMSE) as a measure of efficiency. To predict two-year longitudinal clinical outcomes, the proposed model used predictive modelling with machine learning, with the elastic-net53 and random forest54 algorithms being trained on a combination of clinical variables, inflammatory cytokine measurements and demographic variables (age and gender). Elastic net is a linear regression technique that minimises overfitting by using both L1 and L2 regularisations. R. Mathur et al. [56] proposed various machine learning algorithms to improve the performance of datasets and early prediction of disease at the right time. The accuracy obtained from the combined effect of the KNN algorithm with ANN is greater than that obtained from other algorithms, according to the experimental results.

Ulagamuthalvi et al. [57] proposed a method to provide high accuracy of prediction for the Parkinson's disease dataset using machine learning algorithms. The proposed system used two machine learning algorithms which are logistic regression and XGBoost. The maximum classification rate is achieved by XGBoost than LR with an accuracy of 96%, whereas LR achieved only 79% accuracy. Franz et al. [58] were able to meet the large dataset size requirements by using a supervised data collection method that enabled them to generate detailed annotations in one-minute intervals. To their knowledge, no other large-scale collection of expert annotations on a one-minute basis has been published. Srilatha et al. [59] have presented in the field of computer vision, suggesting that classification is a crucial role. Image classification is the method of categorising images into one of many predefined groups, which include image sensors, image preprocessing, object detection, object segmentation, feature extraction and object classification. For image classification, a variety of techniques have been developed. The highest concentration is on using various classifiers combined with several segmentation algorithms for the detection of tumours using image processing.

Shraddha et al. [60] have proposed performance parameters used by authors, which are true positive, true negative and accuracy. Authors make use of various semi-supervised classifiers for intrusion detection. All classifiers used an NSL KDD dataset for intrusion detection. Mallikarjuna et al. [61] presented the backpropagation approach which compares normality and abnormality using a feedback-based approach. The derived feature sequences of regular and abnormal walking, as well as the three classes A, B, C, D normal, Parkinson's gait, hemiplegic gait and neuropathic gait datasets, were compared with the normal dataset during the training process. Azadeh Mozhdehfarahbakhsh et al. [62] proposed a convolutional neural network and MRI-based deep learning model to predict Parkinson's disease and its stages. In Parkinson's disease, it is always a challenge to identify its stages and its progression. Based on the technical advancements in artificial intelligence, supervised and unsupervised machine learning methods are used on clinical and paraclinical datasets to accurately diagnose PD, identify its stage and predict it. The MRI dataset is used in the proposed model to effectively predict PD and identify its stages. The proposed method produced 94% accuracy at distinguishing the stages. Makarious et al. proposed [63] an automated ML pipeline model to make improved multi-omic forecasts of PD. The multimodel information is utilised in a robotised ML framework to tune the exhibition. The underlying model showed a territory under the bend (AUC) of 89.72% for the analysis of PD. The tuned model was then tried for approval on outer information (PDBP, AUC 85.03%). Joining information modalities beats the single biomarker worldview. The model created improves illness hazard prediction. The proposed framework develops the quality articulation networks for the up-and-coming age of genomics-inferred mediations. Our mechanised ML approach permits complex prescient models to be reproducible and available in the local area.

Afzal Hussain Shahid and Maheshwari Prasad Singh [64] proposed a PCA-based deep neural network (DNN) model to foresee motor-UPDRS and total-UPDRS in Parkinson's disease (PD) movement. The model utilised the decreased info highlight space of Parkinson's telemonitoring dataset for checking the movement. PCA was utilised to extricate the highlights from the entire dataset that incorporate the age and sex of the PD patients. Clinically, age and sex influence the UPDRS score. The model's expectation precision is estimated by wellness boundaries, mean absolute error (MAE), root mean squared error (RMSE) and coefficient of determination (R2). The MAE, RMSE and R2 are 0.926, 1.422 and 0.970 separately for engine UPDRS. These qualities are 1.334, 2.221 and 0.956 separately for total-UPDRS. Atiqur Rahman et al. [65] proposed a PD discovery model by separating cepstral highlights from the voice signs and ordering by support vector machine. To characterise the extricated highlights, the model utilised dimensionality decrease through linear discriminant analysis and did the order by support vector machine. The proposed model is approved and tried with ten diverse AI models. The proposed technique delivered area under curve (AUC) of 88%, affectability of 73.33%, particularity of 84% and additionally, the proposed clever framework was recreated utilising openly accessible various sorts of voice information base. Harshvardhan Tiwari et al. [66] proposed a machine learning model to classify whether a person has Parkinson's disease or not. The six classification algorithms are used for the classification of PD from the UCI Parkinson's disease dataset. The algorithms such as logistic regression, support vector machine (SVM), decision tree, K-nearest neighbour (KNN) and XGBoost (extreme gradient boosting) are used to predict the outcome of whether the person is healthy or Parkinson's disease–affected based on the voice input parameters. The simulation results proved that the ensemble techniques produced 95% accuracy in testing and 100% in training compared to base classification algorithms such as XGBoost, bagging classifier.

I. G. Tsoulos et al. [67] proposed a man-made consciousness framework to separate PD patients from sound volunteers and decide various highlights of the sickness inside a partner of PD subjects. The neural network construction (NNC) strategy was utilised to group information gathered by a portable application (iMotor, Apptomics Inc., Wellesley, MA) into two classifications: PD for patients and HV. The strategy was tried on a progression of information recently gathered, and the outcomes were looked at against more conventional strategies for neural organisation preparing. The NNC calculation segregated individual PD patients from HVs with 93.11% precision and ON versus OFF state with 76.5% precision. Sajal et al. [68] proposed a continuous observing framework with AI ways to deal with distinguishing PD utilising rest quake and vowel phonation information procured by cell phones with built-in accelerometer and voice recorder sensors. The information is principally gathered from analysed PD patients and healthy individuals for building and streamlining AI models that show better accuracy. The information from recently speculated PD patients is gathered, and the prepared calculations are assessed to recognise PD. After discovery, PD recognised patients are associated with a close-by nervous system specialist for a meeting. The framework may refresh the model by retraining it to utilise the most recent information subsequent to accepting patients' criticism analysed by the nervous system specialist. The most elevated exactness in PD location utilising disconnected information was 98.3% from voice information and 98.5% from quake information when utilised independently. In the two cases, K-closest neighbours (kNN) gave the most noteworthy precision over support vector machine (SVM) and naive Bayes (NB). The normal exactness of PD discovery becomes 99.8% when average-gathering was performed on the dominant part vote from kNN, SVM and NB.

D. Ahmadi Rastegar et al. [69] proposed a framework with longitudinally evaluated fringe inflammatory cytokines and utilised AI calculations to decide the relative degree to which the cytokines add to the longitudinal forecast of PD symptomology. It utilised serum tests from a PD patients with and without the regular leucine-rich recurrent kinase 2 (LRRK2) G2019S transformation. The proposed framework is utilised to assess the changeability of fringe inflammatory cytokine levels in people over a one-year time period. Various components may add to the guideline of fringe cytokine levels, and while longitudinal investigations have been directed for some neurodegenerative illnesses, like Alzheimer's disease, longitudinal appraisal of fringe inflammatory cytokines in PD is deficient. Utilising the normalised root mean square error (NRMSE) as a proportion of execution, the best expectation models were for the engine indication seriousness scales, with NRMSE of 0.1123 for the Hoehn and Yahr scale and 0.1193 for the Unified Parkinson's Disease Rating Scale section three (UPDRS III). Luigi Borzì et al. [70] proposed a FOG location calculation utilising wearable frameworks and ML-based order calculations. The framework got the common corruption of the strolling design going before FOG scenes to accomplish dependable FOG prediction utilising AI calculations and confirm

whether dopaminergic treatment influences the capacity of our framework to identify and foresee FOG. A cohort of 11 Parkinson's disease patients getting (on) and
not accepting (off) dopaminergic treatment was furnished with two inertial sensors
set on each shin and requested to play out a coordinated up-and-go test. The progres-
sion-to-step division is performed on the precise speed signals and ensuing element
extraction from both time and recurrence spaces. The proposed framework utilised
a covering approach to include choice and streamlined distinctive AI classifiers to
get FOG and pre-FOG scenes. For pre-FOG discovery, the arrangement calculation
accomplished 84.1% (85.5%) affectability, 85.9% (86.3%) particularity and 85.5%
(86.1%) exactness. At the point when the order model was prepared with information
from patients on (off) and tried on patients off (on), the ML-based characterisation calculation created 84.0% (56.6%) affectability, 88.3% (92.5%) explicitness and
87.4% (86.3%) exactness.

Yulianti et al. [71] proposed a component choice method to anticipate the PD profi-
ciently since the dataset with numerous highlights can expand intricacy, yet not all highlights affect the consequences of the investigation. Immaterial highlights decreased
the model execution. The voice dataset from the UCI archive is utilised in this model.
The dataset is grouped utilising a decision tree arrangement technique. In light of the
reproduction, the decision tree gained 64.17% precision and 0.6417 AUC, the decision
tree with forward determination created 71.74% exactness and 0.7171 AUC and the
decision tree with reverse choice delivered 69.42% precision and 0.6942 AUC.

13.3   PERFORMANCE ANALYSIS

It is observed from Table 13.1 that many authors have proposed systems to improve
the prediction accuracy for Parkinson's disease. Several aspects of PD biomarkers
need to be investigated further. More longitudinal research is required to assess
which biomarker strategies would be most effective in detecting PD earlier and recognising preclinical, at-risk populations. Instead of relying solely on clinical assessment, potential diagnostic imaging or biofluid assays should be compared to the
gold standard in neuropathology, since diagnostic accuracy in some settings may
be poor. Methodologies for biomarker studies must be fine-tuned and standardised,
which is particularly important for biofluid assays and neuroimaging protocols, as
methodological variations may lead to inconsistent results. Last but not least, new
biomarkers and analytical techniques must be discovered. The research of imaging
methods to detect α-synuclein in the brain is underway. Multimodal datasets, such
as those derived from various types of neuroimaging in combination with biofluid
measurements and other data, can help us better understand PD and, through various
models, differentiate PD patients (or at-risk persons) from healthy controls, atypical
parkinsonian syndromes, and other neurodegenerative conditions. It's important to
understand that sensitivity and precision coexist in a healthy way. Increased sensitivity—the ability to accurately recognise individuals who have the disease—is
normally accompanied by a decrease in specificity (meaning more false positives).
Similarly, high specificity—when a test does a decent job of excluding people who
don't have the disease—typically means lower sensitivity (more false negatives).

TABLE 13.1
Performance Analysis of Various Existing Systems

Proposed Algorithm	Features and Dataset Used	Number of Features Selected for Processing	Accuracy (%)
Minimum Redundancy Maximum Relevance feature selection	Speech	20	90.3
Fuzzy C means clustering and pattern recognition	Speech		68.04
Wrapper feature selection scheme			72 to 92
Speech signal processing	Dysphonia	10	99
Artificial neural network	Speech		85.92
Multilayer perceptron (MLP) with backpropagation learning			91.45
Rough set approach	Speech	22	100
Genetic algorithm and SVM	Speech	14	96.06 for 4 optimised features 93.58 for 7 optimised features 93.61 for 9 optimised features
Nested-RF and nested-SVM	Cancer	5	Up to 93
SVM and correlation-based classification	Speech	5	90.5 recognition rate 0.97 AUC
Neural networks, data mining neural analysis and regression analysis	SAS software		92.9, 84.3, 88.6, 84.3
Parallel distributed neural network	Voice		92.9
PCA and DLA	Vision	1	
SPM	Voice	3	85
MFCC	Speech	20	Quantisation result 90 and 95
Regression, decision tree and neural network	Databank		Error probability 5.15, 8.47, 23.7
SVM and RFBNN	Voice	7	RFBNN—91, SVM—83
FKNN-based system	Voice	2	96.07
Data mining and machine learning	Hip	2	92
Naive Bayes FNSB, CFS-NB		4	97
SVM, KNN, PLS and random tree	Voice	3	
Nested-RF and nested-SVM		5	93

(*Continued*)

TABLE 13.1 (CONTINUED)
Performance Analysis of Various Existing Systems

Proposed Algorithm	Features and Dataset Used	Number of Features Selected for Processing	Accuracy (%)
Prediction model tree–based classification	Voice	6	Decision tree—85.08 ID3—75.33 Decision stumps—83.5
Neural networks (ANN), data mining, neural regression and decision tree	Voice	10	96.88
Clonclas and probabilistic neural network	Immunity	3	100
Kernal-based extreme learning machine with subtractive clustering features (SCFWKELM)	Voice	10	99.49
Kernal-based extreme learning machine with subtractive clustering features weighting (CFWKELM)	Voice	10	99.49
SVM, KNN, random forest and naive Bayes	Voice	26	88.9
SVM	Eyes	1	85.48
SVM-L2 norm metric conjunction	Eyes		77
CART, SCM and ANN	Voice	1	93.7
Discretisation method, SVM, C4.5, k-nearest neighbour and naive Bayes	Body movement	28	
Artificial neural network	Neurodegenerative disorders	6	
Multilayer perceptron with backpropagation learning algorithm, RBF, ANN	Voice		MLP—93.22 RBF—86.44
Random forest (RF), SVM, GA-RF, GA-SVM	Voice	4	94
Radial basis function neural network (RBFNN) based on PSO and PCA with LPF	Brain		RFBNN—89.91 PCA + RBFNN—88.92 PCA + PSO + RBFNN—88.92

(Continued)

TABLE 13.1 (CONTINUED)
Performance Analysis of Various Existing Systems

Proposed Algorithm	Features and Dataset Used	Number of Features Selected for Processing	Accuracy (%)
Fuzzy entropy-based feature selection	Voice		Mean accuracy—85.03
Wavelet analysis (using MNN)	Speech		Between 80 and 100
Computer-aided diagnosis (CADs) with CFS algorithm			74.47
Naive Bayes and KNN	Speech		K-nearest neighbour—80 Naïve Bayes—93.3

13.4 CONCLUSION

A similar investigation on ML techniques as far as different execution measurements like particularity, affectability, exactness, ROC, highlight chose and accuracy has been finished. From this investigation, it is noticed that for prediction, discourse and voice have been considered as significant boundaries and have delivered extensive precision. Notwithstanding discourse and voice, utilisation of additional factors like stances, developments and outward appearances can give better outcomes and improve the exactness in diagnosing Parkinson's disease and furthermore to assist the clinical administration with better outcomes to diminish the danger level.

REFERENCES

1. Rubén Armañanzas, Concha Bielza, Kallol Ray Chaudhuri, Pablo Martinez-Martin, and Pedro Larrañaga, "Unveiling Relevant Non-Motor Parkinson's Disease Severity Symptoms Using Machine Learning Approach", *Elsevier Journal of Artificial intelligence in medicine*, vol. 58, no. 3, 2013, pp. 195–202.
2. Zhennao Cai, Jianhua Gu, Caiyun Wen, Dong Zhao, Chunyu Huang, Hui Huang, Changfei Tong, Jun Li, and Huiling Chen, "An Intelligent Parkinson's Disease Diagnostic System Based on a Chaotic Bacterial Foraging Optimization Enhanced Fuzzy KNN Approach", *Computational and Mathematical Methods in Medicine*, vol. 2018, 2018, Article ID 2396952. doi: 10.1155/2018/2396952.
3. L. Salhi, T. Mourad, and A. Cherif, "Voice Disorders Identification Using Multilayer Neural Network", *Pathology*, vol. 2, no. 7, 2008, p. 8.
4. Md. Sakibur Rahman Sajal, Md. Tanvir Ehsan, Ravi Vaidyanathan, Shouyan Wang, Tipu Aziz, and Khondaker Abdullah Al Mamun, "Telemonitoring Parkinson's Disease Using Machine Learning by Combining Tremor and Voice Analysis," *Brain Informatics*, vol. 7, no. 12, 2020, pp. 1–11. doi: 10.1186/s40708-020-00113-1.

5. Tarigoppula V. S. Sriram, M. Venkateswara Rao, G. V. Satya Narayana, D. S. V. G. K. Kaladhar, and T. Pandu Ranga Vital, "Intelligent Parkinson Disease Prediction Using Machine Learning Algorithms", *International Journal of Engineering and Innovative Technology (IJEIT)*, vol. 3, no. 3, 2013, pp. 212–215.

6. Hung Nguyen, Karina Lebel, Sarah Bogard, Etienne Goubault, Patrick Boissy, and Christian Duval, "Using Inertial Sensors to Automatically Detect and Segment Activities of Daily Living in People with Parkinson's Disease", *IEEE Transactions on Neural Systems and Rehabilitation Engineering*, vol. 26, no. 1, January 2018, pp. 197–204.

7. Bruno Andò, Salvatore Baglio, Vincenzo Marletta, Antonio Pistorio, Valeria Dibilio, Giovanni Mostile, Alessandra Nicoletti, and Mario Zappia, "A Wearable Device to Support the Pull Test for Postural Instability Assessment in Parkinson's Disease", *IEEE Transactions on Instrumentation and Measurement*, vol. 67, no. 1, January 2018, pp. 218–228.

8. Alberto Fung, Eugene C. Lai, and Beom-Chan Lee, "Usability and Validation of the Smarter Balance System: An Unsupervised Dynamic Balance Exercises System for Individuals with Parkinson's Disease", *IEEE Transactions on Neural Systems and Rehabilitation Engineering*, vol. 26, no. 4, April 2018, pp. 798–806, doi: 10.1109/TNSRE.2018.2808139.

9. A. H. Hadjahmadi and T. J. Askari, "A Decision Support System for Parkinson's Disease Diagnosis Using Classification and Regression Tree", *The Journal of Mathematics and Computer Science*, vol. 4, no. 2, 2012, pp. 257–263.

10. Ali Saad, Iyad Zaarour, Abbas Zeinedine, Mohammad Ayache, Paul Bejjani, François Guerin, and Dimitri Lefebvre, "A Preliminary Study of the Causality of Freezing of Gait for Parkinson's Disease Patients: Bayesian Belief Network Approach", *International Journal of Computer Science Issues*, vol. 10, no. 2, 2013, pp. 88–95.

11. S. Amit, M. Ashutosh, A. Bhattacharya, and F. Revilla, "Understanding Postural Response of Parkinson's Subjects Using Nonlinear Dynamics and Support Vector Machines", *Austin Journal of Biomedical Engineering*, vol. 1, no. 1, March 2014, p. id1005.

12. Aprajita Sharma and Ram Nivas Giri, "Automatic Recognition of Parkinson's Disease via Artificial Neural Network and Support Vector Machine", *International Journal of Innovative Technology and Exploring Engineering*, vol. 4, no. 3, 2014, pp. 35–41.

13. Arvind Kumar Tiwari, "Machine Learning Based Approaches for Prediction of Parkinson's Disease", *International Journal of Machine Learning and Applications*, vol. 3, no. 2, June 2016, pp. 33–39.

14. Athanasios Tsanas, Max A. Little, Patrick E. McSharry, Jennifer Spielman, and Lorraine O. Ramig, "Novel Speech Signal Processing Algorithms for High Accuracy Classification of Parkinson's Disease", *IEEE Transactions on Biomedical Engineering*, vol. 59, no. 5, 2012, pp. 1264–1271.

15. Austin H. Chen, Chia Hung Lin, and Chih Hung Cheng, "New Approaches to Improve the Performance of Disease Classification Using Nested–Random Forest and Nested–Support Vector Machine Classifiers", *Research Notes in Information Science*, vol. 14, 2013, pp. 587–592.

16. C. Azad, S. Jain, and V. K. Jha, "Design and Analysis of Data Mining Based Prediction Model for Parkinson's Disease", *International Journal of Computer Science Engineering*, vol. 1, no. 1, 2014, pp. 181–189.

17. S. Bouchikhi, A. Boublenza, A. Benosman, and M. A. Chikh, "Parkinson's Disease Detection with SVM Classifier and Relief-F Features Selection Algorithm", *South East Europe Journal of Soft Computing*, vol. 2, no. 1, 2013, pp. 1–4.

18. A. H. Chen, C. H. Cheng, and C. H. Lin, "The Improvement of Parkinson's Disease Classification Using Genetic Algorithm–Random Forests and Genetic Algorithm–Support Vector Machine Methods", *International Journal of Advancements in Computing Technology*, vol. 4, no. 21, 2012.

19. A. H. Chen and C. H. Lin, "Optimizing the Performance of Disease Classification Using Nested-Random Forest and Nested Support Vector Machine Classifiers", *Journal of Chemical & Pharmaceutical Research*, vol. 5, no. 12, 2013, pp. 1521–1528.

20. H. L. Chen, C. C. Huang, X. G. Yu, X. Xu, X. Sun, G. Wang, and S. J. Wang, "An Efficient Diagnosis System for Detection of Parkinson's Disease Using Fuzzy k-Nearest Neighbour Approach", *Expert Systems with Applications*, vol. 40, no. 1, 2013, pp. 263–271.

21. Chien-Wen Cho, Wen-Hung Chao, Sheng-Huang Lin, and You-Yin Chen, "A Vision-Based Analysis System for Gait Recognition in Patients with Parkinson's Disease", *Elsevier Journal of Expert Systems with Applications*, vol. 36, no. 3, 2009, pp. 7033–7039.

22. S. G. Farhad and M. Peyman, "A Case Study of Parkinson's Disease Diagnosis Using Artificial Neural Networks", *International Journal of Computer Applications*, vol. 73, no. 19, 2013, pp. 1748–1760.

23. Z. Cai, J. Gu, and H. Chen, "A New Hybrid Intelligent Framework for Predicting Parkinson's Disease," *IEEE Access*, vol. 5, 2017, pp. 17188–17200. doi: 10.1109/ACCESS.2017.2741521.

24. H. Hazan, D. Hilu, L. Manevitz, L. O. Ramig, and S. Sapir, "Early Diagnosis of Parkinson's Disease via Machine Learning on Speech Data", in *2012 IEEE 27th Convention of Electrical & Electronics Engineers in Israel (IEEEI)*, 2012, pp. 1–4. IEEE.

25. Indira Rustempasic and Mehmet Can, "Diagnosis of Parkinson's Disease Using Fuzzy C-Means Clustering and Pattern Recognition", *South East Europe Journal of Soft Computing*, vol. 2, no. 1, 2013, pp. 42–49.

26. J. Rusz, R. Cmejla, H. Ruzickova, J. Klempir, V. Majerova, J. Picmausova, J. Roth, and E. Ruzicka, "Acoustic Analysis of Voice and Speech Characteristics in Early Untreated Parkinson's Disease", in *7th International Workshop on Models and Analysis of Vocal Emissions for Biomedical Applications*, August 25–27, 2011, pp. 181–184.

27. T. Kapoor and R. K. Sharma, "Parkinson's Disease Diagnosis Using Mel-Frequency Cepstral Coefficients and Vector Quantization", *International Journal of Computer Applications*, vol. 14, no. 3, 2011, pp. 43–46.

28. E. Kaya, O. Findik, I. Babaoglu, and A. Arslan, "Effect of Discretization Method on the Diagnosis of Parkinson's Disease", *International Journal of Innovative Computing, Information and Control*, vol. 7, 2011, pp. 4669–4678.

29. Kenneth Revett, Florin Gorunescu, and Abdel-Badeeh Mohamed Salem, "Feature Selection in Parkinson's Disease: A Rough Sets Approach", in *IEEE International Multiconference on Computer Science and Information Technology (IMCSIT'09)*, October 2009, pp. 425–428.

30. A. Khemphila and V. Boonjing, "Parkinsons Disease Classification Using Neural Network and Feature Selection", World Academy of Science, Engineering and Technology, *International Journal of Mathematical, Computational, Physical, Electrical and Computer Engineering*, vol. 6, no. 4, 2012, pp. 377–380.

31. B. K. Kihel and M. Benyettou, "Parkinson's Disease Recognition Using Artificial Immune System", *Journal of Software Engineering and Applications*, vol. 4, no. 07, 2011, p. 391.

32. Korosh Rouhollahi, Mehran Emadi Andani, Seyed Mahdi Karbassi, and Iman Izadi, "Design of Robust Adaptive Controller and Feedback Error Learning for Rehabilitation in Parkinson's Disease: A Simulation Study", *IET Journal of System Biology*, vol. 11, no. 1, March 2017, pp. 19–29.

33. P. Luukka, "Feature Selection Using Fuzzy Entropy Measures with Similarity Classifier", *Expert Systems with Applications*, vol. 38, no. 4, 2011, pp. 4600–4607.

34. C. Ma, J. Ouyang, H. L. Chen, and X. H. Zhao, "An Efficient Diagnosis System for Parkinson's Disease Using Kernel-Based Extreme Learning Machine with Subtractive Clustering Features Weighting Approach", *Computational and Mathematical Methods in Medicine*, vol. 2014, 2014.

35. Mehmet Can, "Diagnosis of Parkinson's Disease by Boosted Neural Networks", *South East Europe Journal of Soft Computing*, vol. 2, no. 1, March 2013, pp. 7–13.

36. Mehmet Fatih Caglar, Bayram Cetisli, and Inayet Burcu Toprak, "Automatic Recognition of Parkinson's Disease from Sustained Phonation Tests Using ANN and Adaptive Neuro-Fuzzy Classifier", *Journal of Engineering Science and Design*, vol. 1, no. 2, 2010, pp. 59–64.

37. Mohammad Shahbakhi, Danial Taheri Far, and Ehsan Tahami, "Speech Analysis for Diagnosis of Parkinson's Disease Using Genetic Algorithm and Support Vector Machine", *Journal of Biomedical Science and Engineering*, vol. 7, 2014, pp. 147–156. doi: 10.4236/jbise.2014.74019.

38. D. A. Morales, Y. Vives-Gilabert, B. Gómez-Ansón, E. Bengoetxea, P. Larrañaga, C. Bielza, and M. Delfino, "Predicting Dementia Development in Parkinson's Disease Using Bayesian Network Classifiers", *Psychiatry Research: NeuroImaging*, vol. 213, no. 2, 2013, 92–98.

39. Resul Das, "A Comparison of Multiple Classification Methods for Diagnosis of Parkinson Disease", *Elsevier Journal of Expert Systems with Applications*, vol. 37, no. 2, 2010, pp. 1568–1572.

40. C. Nivedita, A. Yogender, and R. K. Sinha, "Artificial Neural Network Based Classification of Neurodegenerative Diseases", *Advances in Biomedical Engineering Research (ABER)*, vol. 1, no. 1, 2013.

41. A. Ozcift and A. Gulten, "Classifier Ensemble Construction with Rotation Forest to Improve Medical Diagnosis Performance of Machine Learning Algorithms", *Computer Methods and Programs in Biomedicine*, vol. 104, no. 3, 2011, pp. 443–451.

42. R. Prashanth, S. D. Roy, P. K. Mandal, and S. Ghosh, "Parkinson's Disease Detection Using Olfactory Loss and REM Sleep Disorder Features", in *2014 36th Annual International Conference of the IEEE in Engineering in Medicine and Biology Society (EMBC)*, 2014, pp. 5764–5767. IEEE.

43. A. W. Przybyszewski, "Applying Data Mining and Machine Learning Algorithms to Predict Symptom Development in Parkinson's Disease", *Annales Academiae Medicae Silesiensis*, vol. 68, no. 5, 2014, pp. 332–349.

44. R. Geetha Ramani and G. Sivagami, "Parkinson Disease Classification Using Data Mining Algorithms", *International Journal of Computer Applications*, vol. 32, no. 9, 2011, pp. 17–22.

45. R. N. Alcalay, E. Caccappolo, H. Mejia-Santana, M.-X. Tang, L. Rosado, M. Orbe Reilly, D. Ruiz, B. Ross, M. Verbitsky, S. Kisselev, E. Louis, C. Comella, A. Colcher, D. Jennings, M. Nance, S. Bressman, W. K. Scott, C. Tanner, S. Mickel, H. Andrews, C. Waters, S. Fahn, L. Cote, S. Frucht, B. Ford, M. Rezak, K. Novak, J. H. Friedman, R. Pfeiffer, L. Marsh, B. Hiner, A. Siderowf, H. Payami, E. Molho, S. Factor, R. Ottman, L. N. Clark, and K. Marder, "Cognitive performance of GBA mutation carriers with early-onset PD: the CORE-PD study", *Neurology*, vol. 78, no. 18, May 2012, pp. 1434–1440. doi: 10.1212/WNL.0b013e318253d54b.

46. A. Saad, I. Zaarour, P. Bejjani, and M. Ayache, "Handwriting and Speech Prototypes of Parkinson Patients: Belief Network Approach", *International Journal of Computer Science Issues*, vol. 9, 2012.

47. C. Salvatore, A. Cerasa, I. Castiglioni, F. Gallivanone, A. Augimeri, M. Lopez, and A. Quattrone, "Machine Learning on Brain MRI Data for Differential Diagnosis of Parkinson's Disease and Progressive Supranuclear Palsy", *Journal of Neuroscience Methods*, vol. 222, 2014, pp. 230–237. doi: 10.1016/j.jneumeth.2013.11.016. Epub 2013 Nov 26. PMID: 24286700.

48. V. Sellam and J. Jagadeesan, "Classification of Normal and Pathological Voice Using SVM and RBFNN", *Journal of Signal and Information Processing*, vol. 2014, 2014.

49. Tobias Bocklet, Elmar Nöth, and Georg Stemmer, "Detection of Persons with Parkinson's Disease by Acoustic, Vocal, and Prosodic Analysis", in *IEEE Workshop on Automatic Speech Recognition and Understanding (ASRU)*, 11–15, December 2011, pp. 478–483.

50. A. Tsanas, M. A. Little, P. E. McSharry, and L. O. Ramig, "Nonlinear Speech Analysis Algorithms Mapped to a Standard Metric Achieve Clinically Useful Quantification of Average Parkinson's Disease Symptom Severity", *Journal of the Royal Society Interface*, vol. 8, no. 59, 2010, pp. 842–855.

51. X. Wan, C. Yang, Q. Yang, et al., "MegaSNPHunter: A Learning Approach to Detect Disease Predisposition SNPs and High Level Interactions in Genome Wide Association Study", *BMC Bioinformatics*, vol. 10, 2009, p. 13. doi: 10.1186/1471-2105-10-13.

52. D. Wu, K. Warwick, Z. Ma, M. N. Gasson, J. G. Burgess, S. Pan, and T. Z. Aziz, "Prediction of Parkinson's Disease Tremor Onset Using a Radial Basis Function Neural Network Based on Particle Swarm Optimization", *International Journal of Neural Systems*, vol. 20, no. 2, 2010, pp. 109–116.

53. I. Mandal and N. Sairam, "New Machine-Learning Algorithms for Prediction of Parkinson's Disease", *International Journal of Systems Science*, vol. 45, no. 3, 2014, pp. 647–666. doi: 10.1080/00207721.2012.724114.

54. G. Pahuja and T. N. Nagabhushan, "A Comparative Study of Existing Machine Learning Approaches for Parkinson's Disease Detection", *IETE Journal of Research*, vol. 67, no. 1, 2018, pp. 4–14. doi: 10.10 80/ 03772063.2018.1531730.

55. Diba Ahmadi Rastegar, Nicholas Ho, Glenda M. Halliday, and Nicolas Dzamko, "Parkinson's Progression Prediction Using Machine Learning and Serum Cytokines", *Nature Partnering Journal Parkinson's Disease*, vol. 5, no. 14, 2019, pp. 1–8. doi: 10.1038/s41531-019-0086-4.

56. R. Mathur, V. Pathak, and D. Bandil, "Parkinson Disease Prediction Using Machine Learning Algorithm", in Rathore, V., Worring, M., Mishra, D., Joshi, A., and Maheshwari, S. (eds), *Emerging Trends in Expert Applications and Security. Advances in Intelligent Systems and Computing*, vol. 841, 2019, Springer, Singapore. doi: 10.1007/978-981-13-2285-3_42.

57. V. Ulagamuthalvi, G. Kulanthaivel, G. S. N. Reddy, and G. Venugopal, "Identification of Parkinson's Disease Using Machine Learning Algorithms", *Bioscience Biotechnology. Research Communications*, vol. 13, no. 2, 2020. doi: 10.21786/bbrc/13.2/32.

58. M. Franz, J. Pfister, T. Taewoong, and U. D. C. Pichler, "High-Resolution Motor State Detection in Parkinson's Disease Using Convolutional Neural Networks", *Scientific Reports*, vol. 10, 2020, pp. 58–60.

59. K. Srilatha and V. Ulagamuthalvi, "A Comparative Study on Tumor Classification Research", *Journal of Pharmacy and Technology*, vol. 12, no. 1, 2019, pp. 407–411.

60. S. Khonde and V. Ulagamuthalvi, "Fusion of Feature Selection and Random Forest for an Anomaly Based Intrusion Detection System", *Journal of Computational and Theoretical Nanoscience*, vol. 16, 2019, pp. 3603–3607.

61. Mallikarjuna B. R. Viswanathan and Bharat Bhushan Naib, "Feedback-Based Gait Identification Using Deep Neural Network Classification", *Journal of Critical Reviews*, vol. 7, 2020, pp. 661–667.

62. Azadeh Mozhdehfarahbakhsh, Saman Chitsazian, Prasun Chakrabarti, Tulika Chakrabarti, Babak Kateb, and Mohammad Nami, "An MRI-Based Deep Learning Model to Predict Parkinson's Disease Stages", preprint from *medRxiv*, February 2021. doi: 10.1101/2021.02.19.21252081.

63. Mary B. Makarious, et al., "Multi-Modality Machine Learning Predicting Parkinson's Disease", preprint from *bioRXiv*, March 2021. doi: 10.1101/2021.03.05.434104.

64. Afzal Hussain Shahid and Maheshwari Prasad Singh, "A Deep Learning Approach for Prediction of Parkinson's Disease Progression", *Biomedical Engineering Letters*, vol. 10, 2020, pp. 227–239. doi: 10.1007/s13534-020-00156-7.

65. N. Bhargava, S. Sharma, R. Purohit, and P. S. Rathore, "Prediction of Recurrence Cancer Using J48 Algorithm," in *2017 2nd International Conference on Communication and Electronics Systems (ICCES)*, Coimbatore, 2017, pp. 386–390. doi: 10.1109/CESYS.2017.8321306.

66. Atiqur Rahman, Sanam Shahla Rizvi, Aurangzeb Khan, Aaqif Afzaal Abbasi, Shafqat Ullah Khan, and Tae-Sun Chung, "Parkinson's Disease Diagnosis in Cepstral Domain Using MFCC and Dimensionality Reduction with SVM Classifier", *Mobile Information Systems*, vol. 2021, March 2021, pp. 1–10. doi: 10.1155/2021/8822069.

67. Harshvardhan Tiwari, Shiji K. Shridhar, Preeti V. Patil, K. R. Sinchana, and G. Aishwarya, "Early Prediction of Parkinson's Disease Using Machine Learning and Deep Learning Approaches", *EasyChair*, preprint, January 2021.

68. R. Raturi and A. Kumar, "An Analytical Approach for Health Data Analysis and Finding the Correlations of Attributes Using Decision Tree and W-Logistic Modal Process", *IJIRCCE*, vol. 7, no. 6, 2019, ISSN (Online): 2320-9801 ISSN (Print): 23209798.

69. S. Chandrasekaran and A. Kumar, "Implementing Medical Data Processing with Ann with Hybrid Approach of Implementation", *Journal of Advanced Research in Dynamical and Control Systems – JARDCS*, vol. 10, 2018, pp. 45–52, ISSN-1943-023X.

70. I. G. Tsoulos, G. Mitsi, A. Stavrakoudis, and S. Papapetropoulos , "Application of Machine Learning in a Parkinson's Disease Digital Biomarker Dataset Using Neural Network Construction (NNC) Methodology Discriminates Patient Motor Status", *Frontiers in ICT*, vol. 6, 2019, p. 10. doi: 10.3389/fict.2019.00010.

71. Md. Sakibur Rahman Sajal, Md. Tanvir Ehsan, Ravi Vaidyanathan, Shouyan Wang, Tipu Aziz, and Khondaker Abdullah Al Mamun, "Telemonitoring Parkinson's Disease Using Machine Learning by Combining Tremor and Voice Analysis", *Brain Informatics*, vol. 7, no. 12, 2020, pp. 1–11. doi: 10.1186/s40708-020-00113-1.

Index

For Product Safety Concerns and Information please contact our EU
representative GPSR@taylorandfrancis.com
Taylor & Francis Verlag GmbH, Kaufingerstraße 24, 80331 München, Germany

www.ingramcontent.com/pod-product-compliance
Lightning Source LLC
Chambersburg PA
CBHW060405220326
41598CB00023B/3022